'There has never been a more important time in nu...... control of your own health. We are exposed to literally tens of thousands of chemicals on a daily basis that humans have never been exposed to before ... Low Tox Life is your handbook to making informed choices about reducing your exposure. Alexx provides sensible, achievable and affordable solutions to help you build resilience and be the best you can be.'

DR RON EHRLICH, HOLISTIC HEALTH ADVOCATE, DENTIST, AUTHOR

'This beautiful book identifies many of the man-made toxins that can cause adverse health effects, and provides lots of practical and easy-to-follow tips on how to reduce your exposure.'

NICOLE BIJLSMA, ENVIRONMENTAL MEDICINE EXPERT, PHD CANDIDATE

'This is just the book you need to show you that with a few simple and delicious changes, you can move beyond surviving and indeed, thrive.'

JUDE BLEREAU, WHOLEFOOD CHEF, AUTHOR AND TEACHER

'Low Tox Life is a comprehensive, inspirational and, most importantly, do-able guide to a healthy, low tox life. It's a book you'll certainly come back to time and time again.'

GEORGIA HARDING, NATUROPATH

'Future generations will shake their heads in disbelief at the damage we have done to our only home, and ourselves, in these last two centuries ... They'll also be thankful that the tide turned when courageous spirits like Alexx spoke up and reminded everyone there's a better way forward.'

MARK J. HENRY, FOUNDER AND DEVELOPMENT ENGINEER SOLIDTEKNICS

This book is dedicated to my son,
Sebastien. Everything I do, I do in
my best efforts to try to create a
better world for you, my beautiful.
A world that rewards what's good
and true over what's shiny and
new, and a world that respects
the greatest giver of life to us all –
Mother Nature. May we feed her
well so that she can continue to
feed us well in the circle of life.

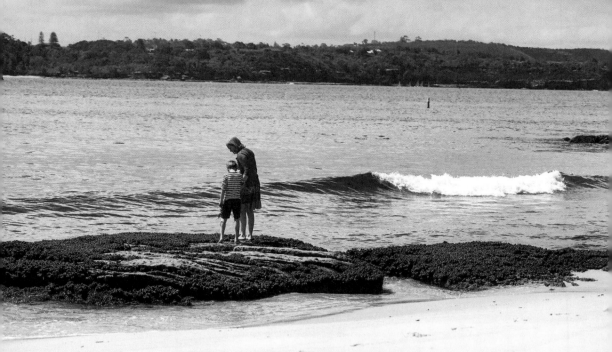

LOW TOX LIFE

A HANDBOOK FOR A HEALTHY YOU AND A HAPPY PLANET

ALEXX STUART

MURDOCH BOOKS

SYDNEY · LONDON

CONTENTS

INTRODUCTION:
SO THERE'S THIS GIRL
I KNOW ...

She eats microwaved popcorn. It seems to make her cough.
She doesn't wonder about that, though. Yummy!

* Her idea of a quick meal is the kind where you pour the contents of
  a sachet into a bowl, add skim milk and microwave for 3 minutes and
  50 seconds on high, and add some chopped zucchini at the last minute.
* She smokes a lot. Nearly a pack a day. She 'really enjoys it' so she's
  not quitting any time soon, although she promised her family with some
  pie-in-the-sky future date she would.
* She has a couple of cocktails or wines after work every night, and
  sometimes a couple of shots of tequila too.
* She's on four different long-term medications for sinus issues,
  contraception and migraine relief.
* She feels nervous if there are no extra-strength painkillers in the house.
  She's not sure why she gets so sick all the time and needs to pop so
  many painkillers and cold and flu tablets. She doesn't really have time
  to think about that. Off to work.
* She gets put on antibiotics every other month for her crappy tonsils,
  and then antifungal medication to deal with the aftermath.
* Her favourite naughty chips are smoky barbecue corn chips. So strange,
  but she coughs and coughs when she eats them and gets a headache.
  But. They. Taste. So. Good.

LOW TOX LIFE

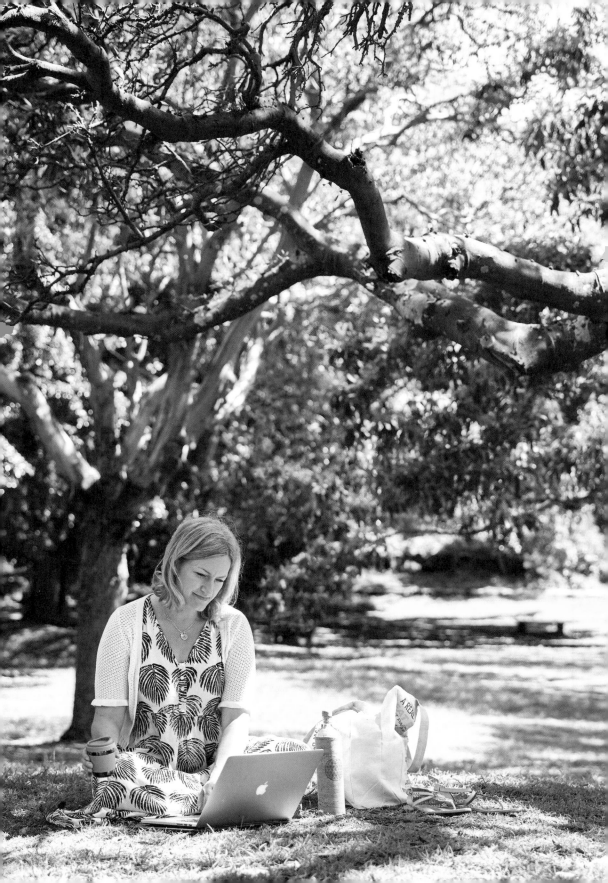

* She has a collection of more than 50 perfumes. And constant headaches. She smells good, though. A fragrance for every mood!

* She uses a strong-smelling aerosol deodorant and has more than 50 skincare products in her cupboards. She uses a scrub with magical micro-exfoliating beads – thousands of them in every tube. She's pretty sure there are fewer wrinkles on her face because of it, just like the ad said, so she raves about it to her friends.

* She has more than 200 make-up items she keeps in a three-tiered display chest. Her eyes water for a couple of hours after doing her face in the mornings and feel a little itchy. Nice colours, though!

* She buys low-fat yoghurt, low-fat dressing, low-fat cottage cheese, low-fat crackers, fat-free chocolate pudding, low-fat tasty cheese, skim milk, fat-free marshmallows and low-fat breakfast-shake poppers as part of her regular shop, all of which she believes are the better choice – because the ads said so, right?

* She uses an air deodoriser so her hospitality uniform is nice and fresh, and fabric softener to make everything super-soft and smell 'yummy'.

* She's really thin, so she must be pretty healthy, right?

'She' could be any one of us out there and probably is, at least in part. But in this case, 'she' is actually me, aged 26.

MY TURNING POINT

• • • • • •

Back then, I was about to have my first encounter with a naturopath – Christine – during a health crisis of a triple round of super-heavy antibiotics that weren't killing my strep throat. I had hit such a low, low point – with so many painkillers for all the headaches, and antibiotics for all the bouts of tonsillitis – that it finally forced me to think outside the box. As a smart person once said, doing the same thing over and over again but expecting a different result is indeed insanity, is it not? Christine changed my life.

The year after that, my boyfriend at the time, now my husband, would be strong enough to quit smoking alongside me and, over the next few years, learn about additives, preservatives and factory farming. We cleaned up our food, reduced chemicals in our home, and brought a gorgeous boy into the world to become a family. All on a peanuts budget, I might add, and as regular people with lots of stuff to get done each day.

Instagram would have us believe that in order to lower our toxic load and live a peaceful life, with simpler food and home products, we need to be full-time homesteaders with unlimited access to funds for perfect linen, rare jars and ceramics, and whitewashed wood; and a knack for arranging flowers and using a sewing machine. And while I may have had access to incredible ceramics for the photos in this book and adore following the lives of people who are fluent in the art of homemaking, I'm rather glad Instagram wasn't around when I first started, because I might have given up, thinking I could never do it all so beautifully. Want to feel the gifts of imperfection on your journey? Follow me there. You'll feel you're doing just fine!

The aim of this game isn't perfection.

If you're busy, messy, tight on budget, and not yet particularly adept at cooking, basket-weaving or making your own salves and balms, *Hello!* There are millions of us out there, and we can still go low tox (more on this soon) in our own way and get really good at it. I've surprised myself by devising idiot-proof recipes, and super-simple ways you can cook and look like a genius to your friends and family! I honestly pinch myself when I think about how I teach people to cook now, when at age 30 I couldn't roast a chicken.

And before you think I'm absolved from all high tox sinning now, and drink multiple green smoothies while doing yoga on a hill at sunset before mixing up ten DIY recipes effortlessly and then doing a meditation practice for an hour before bed, I'm sorry to disappoint, but I'm not perfect. As I type this, I'm drinking a lovely Californian small-batch gin on the rocks. I got my hair coloured yesterday, and because of writing this book, I've not done anything more than a couple of quick sun salutes a day in the last month. The aim of this game isn't perfection. Perfection doesn't exist, and gosh it made me so very happy to come to the realisation that what I'm doing is enough, as long as I'm doing my best.

MAKING CHANGE EASY

• • • • • •

Something I've also come to realise is that while you can't choose a different past, you can always rewrite the rest of *your* book, and that rewrite can be your own. When I was growing up, 1980s and 1990s icons were always trying to force militant change upon me with strict diets and exercise plans, but I always felt I was failing before I began. On *this* journey of change, though – the one I created for myself – I found a lightness, a freedom and an ease. I made my own plan that worked for me and my family and life.

> *On* this *journey of change, though, I found a lightness, a freedom and an ease.*

I want that for you, too. I would hate to think of someone reading this book with a sense of 'not doing it right', so it's important that we look at making a success of change, because I found that the changes I made on this low tox road *stuck* for once. And it was almost always really easy. How could that be when, like most of us, I'd always found making changes so difficult? After a lot of thinking, I now believe that when we make changes that don't stick, it's for any or all of these six reasons:

1. We don't fully understand *why* the change in question is needed.
2. We don't fully understand *how* to make the change effectively.
3. The change we make feels less good than the way things used to be, so it's inevitable that we don't want to stay 'changed' forever – hello to why no strict diet ever actually works in the long term! In the end, the chocolate will win. It always does.
4. We exhaust our mental, financial or time-taking capacity to effect changes – however good they are – and we abandon ship, fast, because the sense of failure is too shameful.
5. We try changing because someone *else* thinks it's a good idea, but we're not quite there yet ourselves.
6. We copy someone else's version of change and we lose ourselves in the process. And then one day we wake up, we think 'I can't do this any more', and we give up.

Once I figured out *why* change hadn't worked in the past, I knew what I needed to do to really make the changes stick – changes that *I* wanted to make and *I* knew were a good idea. Let's look at the six YES factors for positive change, so we're not left with the negatives above:

1. I fully understand why this change is needed.
2. I fully understand the options for how I can make this change.
3. This change feels good, and I'm using a healthy level of guilt, now that I know what I know, to springboard me to upping my game and doing what *I* want to do.
4. I've prioritised the brain space, budget and time to make this change.
5. I don't care what anyone else is doing. *I* think this is a good idea and worth prioritising.
6. I've seen a few different ways to go about it, but this is the way that resonates with me. I'm going to make it my own.

Take plastic bags, for example. In the past, I was aware that plastic bags were polluting our world, but I didn't really understand the full extent of the plastic pollution issue. There was no real fire in my belly. Plastic bags were soooo convenient. Couple that with the fact that I hadn't figured out a way to remember the reusable bags every time I went to the supermarket – which made me a veritable 'sometimes good girl'. When I was tired at the end of a long day's work, I just said yes to the darn bag, okay? So how did I change my habit? By ticking those six YES factors and actually making the change stick. How did I do that? Six ways:

1. I educated myself. I watched a couple of sobering documentaries about single-use plastics that really hit home for me. The fire was in my belly. I fully understood the extent of the issue and was suitably horrified.

2. I made rules. I thought about how I could break the habit of saying yes to a bag and a way of mostly remembering my reusable bags. I set myself a simple *non-negotiable* challenge: if I forgot my reusable bag, I had to either carry the items or leave them there. I started to ensure, quick smart, that this wasn't going to happen often – by leaving reusable bags everywhere: by the front door instead of packed away after putting away the shopping, in the car, in my handbag …

3. I made it bigger than me. I focused on the beauty of the change I was making, for my own sense of accomplishment and for our beautiful planet. I thought of the world my son was inheriting.

4. I made mental space for this change. I chose it as a priority to focus on.

5. I did it because I wanted to. Not just because I 'should'.

6. I did it *my waaaaayyyyy*. Thanks, Frank.

Finally, no more plastic bags.

So rather than change meaning deprivation and hardship, I turned it into a feeling of winning and discovery, across all aspects of the Low Tox Life. I coined that term back in 2012, when I decided to start sharing my experiences, learning and offering others a helping hand along the way.

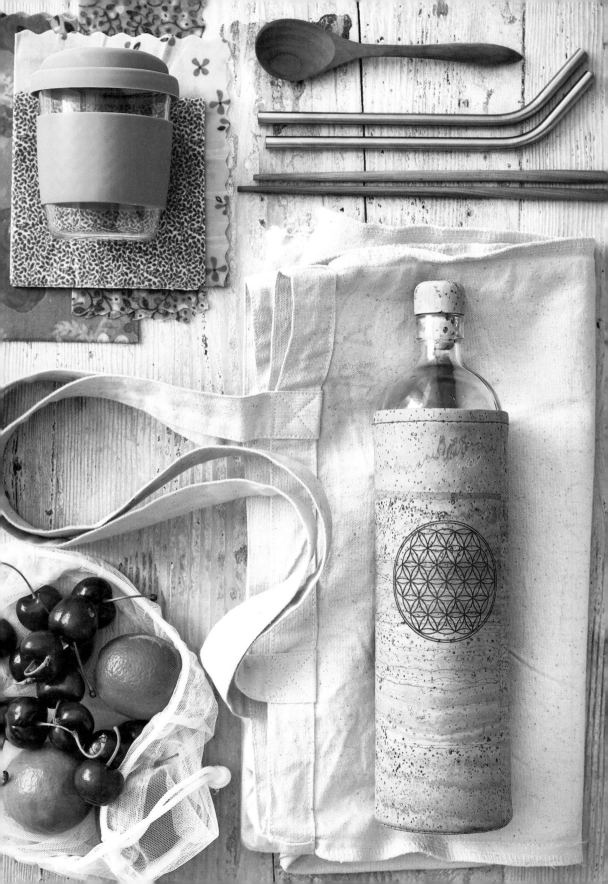

It was *so* easy. I didn't yearn for that processed chocolate bar any more. It actually became a case of 'As If I'd eat that!' rather than 'Oooh, I shouldn't/I can't'. The latter is just not sustainable, and if you find yourself wanting to make changes but still approaching them from a place of 'Ooh, I shouldn't', then you've still got good work to do to make your desired changes stick with more than just guilt. Guilt can be positive if used as a springboard rather than somewhere to wallow, but it's still not enough.

FINDING YOUR OWN REASON TO CHANGE

• • • • • •

Given we're going to be talking about lowering our toxic load in this book, why not ask yourself now: 'Why am I here?' Get in touch with why this topic interests you. Is it for your own personal health gain? Is it the environmental aspect? Is it looking at your baby girl or boy and thinking, 'I just don't want to bring them up in a world of synthetics and excess'? Is there illness in your family that nothing else seems to fix, and you want to explore the potential impact of lowering your toxic load? Is it because you simply want to swap your daily products with ones that will give you peace of mind?

Once you're in touch with a powerful main driver to get you going, you might find that others unfold along the way as you learn new things. Really, though, we all start from one little inkling on some level that this is all worth looking into.

My first reason to do some digging was not being able to handle another day of raging tonsils. My second was my sore gut and swollen glands, which nothing seemed to fix until I tried removing gluten from my diet. Darn it, that was it! My third was my baby boy and wanting to scrutinise and understand everything I was going to put on him and feed him. I'll never forget standing in a supermarket aisle and having one of those Hollywood-movie moments where the actor starts screaming a single high-pitched scream, and to convey how loud the scream is and how big the moment, the camera pans out to surrounding buildings, then the cityscape, then the bird's-eye view, then space – you know those ones? That was me, having 'that moment' as I stood there trying to decipher creams and food pots and thinking: 'What on earth is *in* all this stuff and how did it get there?'

My fourth is to play a bigger game, raise my voice and help as many people as I can to create change at the grassroots. My skin isn't thick enough for policy-making, swinging off boats in the Pacific or organising rallies. If I tried to effect change in those ways, I'd be denying who I was as a person. I'd be doing it *their* way, but that isn't *my* way (to which my friends keep saying 'yet', but we shall see!). And so I've wholeheartedly launched myself into being a gentle activist from my shopping basket, from my kitchen and my home, and out to you and our low tox community. And the beautiful thing is, once you learn all this stuff, it will be your turn to decide what to make of it, how to apply it, and at what speed and to what degree – whether that's by making a few beautiful swaps in your own life and pointing your friends to resources when they ask, or by driving policy change ... We're all needed. All our ways of making a difference matter. The collective is only as powerful as its diversity, after all.

> *All our ways of making a difference matter. The collective is only as powerful as its diversity, after all.*

What it all boils down to us doing in our own sweet way is this: if you're here, it's because you're curious about living more in line with nature through our daily choices of what we put *on* us and *in* us, and choose to have *around* us. The more you learn, the greater your awareness will become of our collective power to create positive influences on our health – and the planet's. You care about the food you buy or grow, and making the best choices possible for people's and the planet's health. You have an awareness about what you're using on your skin, in your cleaning and around your home, and making the best possible choices for people and the planet. You're aware of what you allow your mind to take on and express, and make the best possible choices for happiness, kindness and peace. Am I describing utopian humanity? Why, yes, I believe I am.

Now, conventional black-and-white thinking might have you saying to yourself: 'Why "low" tox rather than "no" tox? That's because I wanted to design a space for myself – and for those I was welcoming in to the low tox community – that wasn't one of extremes and black-and-whites. I recognise that you're going to have a crappy day when you want to think anything *but* peaceful thoughts. You're going to have a juice in a foreign airport and forget your reusable cup or forget to say, 'No straw, please.' You're going to have the lovingly made non-organic, genetically modified grain-fed steak at a friend's place with packet gravy mix. You're going to have a processed biscuit at a morning tea. You're going to receive an online order that's wrapped a thousand times in bubble wrap (seriously, what's with that, though? Write them an email!).

Nothing is black and white. No one can be 'toxin-free' or '100 per cent organic' in today's world. And in my experience – because I did give the extreme a red-hot go for a minute there – it was stressful and I was sour. And frankly, I'm pretty sure that the stress wiped out any of the health benefits, because stress is the silent killer that will undo us all far faster than a non-organic leaf of lettuce ever could. So 'low tox' made it feel achievable, along the way incorporating more and more wonderful changes across body, home, food and mind, without feeling like we'd failed if we weren't perfect. As it turns out, it resonated with thousands, so here we all are, with you now joining us too. Yay!

YOU CAN DO IT

• • • • • •

If you've just embarked on this journey, you have to start somewhere. It's kind of like moving house and thinking 'How am I ever going to pack up this whole apartment?' The answer? One drawer, one cupboard shelf and one toy box at a time. Going low tox is no different. It starts with a deodorant swap or a switch to organic broccoli. From me baring all back there, you can see I began with a fair bit of work to do. There's still work to do now. We're never done, and I find comfort in the fact that we don't have to 'arrive' somewhere and say, 'I'm done. It's perfect now.' There's only doing a little better as you learn better or as funds become available or you have the time to prioritise something. There's no judgement here. Leave any feelings of guilt about what you didn't know in the past at the door and get excited about what's to come. Don't worry about what happens the odd time. Just focus on reaching for awesomeness in what you do *most of the time*.

> AT THE END OF THE DAY THIS IS A BIT LIKE LEARNING A NEW LANGUAGE. YOU'RE NOT GOING TO BE FLUENT IN A WEEK.

You'll become a better and better detective as time goes on. You'll find it easier to make better choices. You'll find beautiful, authentic products and shops that you can trust, and you'll so love the peace you find from knowing where your dollars are going. You'll also find you need less.

There'll always be someone who knows more than you. There'll always be someone who knows less. Don't give yourself a hard time, and don't give anyone else a hard time for only being at the beginning of the journey. Remember that you were there once too.

To go low tox is a very personal thing. I've had people do my courses who end up tree-changing and living in self-built tiny houses after leaving big jobs with multinationals (and yes, for a brief moment when I've seen their amazing stories in our alumni chat groups, I've thought, 'Far out, I'm not doing enough!' And then quickly pulled my attitude into line. That is *their* story, mine is mine. Yours will be yours). Others, though, have just been grateful to make some simple swaps around the home and in daily life, to just feel like they're doing the best for their bustling urban family and their bit for the planet at the same time – and that's 100 per cent okay too.

However the change-making unfolds for you as you explore what's on the pages that follow, know that there's no single picture of success. This is a journey of awakening and curiosity, towards better choices for ourselves and the planet. The way we choose to live our conscious life with the knowledge we acquire? Well, that's entirely up to each of us.

THE CHANGE WE ALL NEED

· · · · · ·

Change has to feel good. It can be challenging, sure, but to be sustainable, it has to feel good. And so I've inadvertently made it my job to help people explore change in their own lives, when it comes to being curious about how and why to lower their daily toxic load and get closer to nature in this busy modern world, and then helping them go about doing that practically – for their body, home, food and mind. To that end, I'd love to welcome you officially to this book – a bit of a bumper starter pack, if you will – on how to live a low tox life.

> *Change has to feel good. It can be challenging, sure, but to be sustainable, it has to feel good.*

Let me leave you with this exciting and powerful thought, called the seventh-generation principle, from the Great Law of Peace, the oral constitution of the Iroquois Confederacy, the oldest living participatory democracy on earth:

> 'IN OUR EVERY DELIBERATION, WE MUST CONSIDER THE IMPACT OF OUR DECISIONS ON THE NEXT SEVEN GENERATIONS.'

(Thank you to the wonderful Native Americans. They sure were onto something.)

Imagine what our choices look like with this phrase as our barometer. A little different from what's all around us now, right?

To start, let's look at making sure you feel empowered all along the way, with a few words on the discovery mindset, and on convenience, on being the first change-maker in your circle, and negotiating the complicated world of 'greenwashing'.

Happy reading and journeying!

CHAPTER ONE

·······

LOW TOX
LIFE

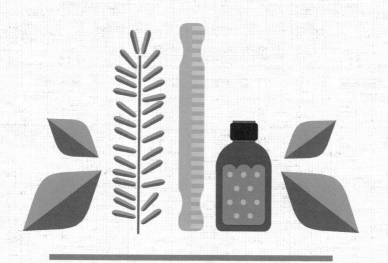

TODAY: THE PERFECT DAY TO GO LOW TOX

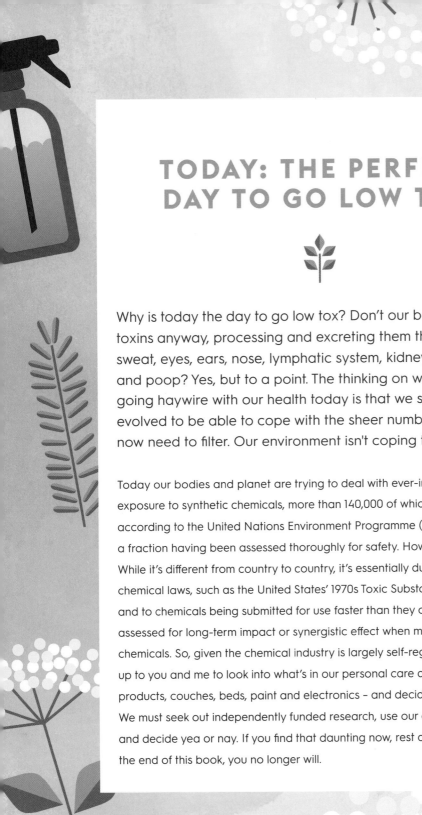

Why is today the day to go low tox? Don't our bodies deal with toxins anyway, processing and excreting them through our sweat, eyes, ears, nose, lymphatic system, kidneys, liver, pee and poop? Yes, but to a point. The thinking on why so much is going haywire with our health today is that we simply haven't evolved to be able to cope with the sheer number of toxins we now need to filter. Our environment isn't coping too well, either.

Today our bodies and planet are trying to deal with ever-increasing exposure to synthetic chemicals, more than 140,000 of which are in circulation, according to the United Nations Environment Programme (UNEP), with only a fraction having been assessed thoroughly for safety. How is that possible? While it's different from country to country, it's essentially due to outdated chemical laws, such as the United States' 1970s Toxic Substances Control Act, and to chemicals being submitted for use faster than they can be adequately assessed for long-term impact or synergistic effect when mixed with other chemicals. So, given the chemical industry is largely self-regulated, it's really up to you and me to look into what's in our personal care and cleaning products, couches, beds, paint and electronics – and decide for ourselves. We must seek out independently funded research, use our critical thinking and decide yea or nay. If you find that daunting now, rest assured that by the end of this book, you no longer will.

Whether or not you've been affected directly yet by the increase in toxins in our world, there's plenty of evidence to suggest that something about our rapid increase in chemical production and use in the past few decades has hurt us, our fellow creatures and the planet in many ways. When we breathe, we're breathing in information; when we eat, we're eating information; when we lather on a body cream, our skin is drinking in information. By design, our beautiful bodies can compute much of what we're feeding them, but what they can't compute causes problems like mixed messages, chemical storage in fat tissues and bacterial imbalances in our gut.

All going low tox really is, is getting back to a place where the information we're feeding our bodies and mind once again makes sense to the human body and the planet around us, so that the information exchange allows us and our planet to thrive, not falter.

SOME BAD NEWS

• • • • • •

Here are a few sobering facts to bear in mind:

* According to the Ocean Cleanup research team, more than 5 trillion pieces of plastic currently litter our oceans.

* In the 1970s and 1980s, about one in 2000 children had autism. Today, the US Centers for Disease Control and Prevention (CDC) estimates that one in 68 eight-year-olds in the United States has an autism spectrum disorder (ASD). In November 2015, the US National Health Statistics Report indicated that one in 45 children across the United States had been diagnosed with an ASD.

* Microbeads found in toothpastes, scrubs, household cleaners and soaps act like tiny magnets for pollutants, capable of concentrating these substances up to 1 million times. Every day, 8 trillion of these tiny plastic beads enter the waterways of the United States alone.

* One in five of us is experiencing a mental illness in any given year in Australia and the United States. In the United Kingdom it's one in four of us. Folks, this ain't normal!

* Reports from several countries state that sperm counts in men have decreased 50 per cent since 1940, and as many as one in six couples finds it difficult to conceive.

* In 2014–15, a staggering 63.4 per cent of Australian adults were overweight or obese – well over half the nation's population. That's almost two in three adults. This is an increase from the 1995 figure of 56.3 per cent, illustrating that the problem is getting worse.

* Approximately 2.5 million tonnes (5.6 billion pounds) of pesticides are used worldwide each year. The current incarnations of the commonly used pesticides contain ingredients and compounds that are endocrine-disruptive (i.e. fiddle around with our natural hormone signalling) and possibly carcinogenic.

* In the past decade, Australia, New Zealand, the United Kingdom and the United States have all seen sharp rises in painkiller use.

* Currently, nine in ten deaths in Australia have chronic disease as an underlying cause. Cardiovascular diseases (coronary heart disease and stroke), dementia and Alzheimer's disease, lung cancer and chronic lower respiratory disease are the most common of these causes, together responsible for 40 per cent of all deaths. What ever happened to dying of old age?

* According to the US Environmental Protection Agency, 15.1 million tons of textile waste was generated in 2013, of which 12.8 million tons were discarded. On average we each throw out 30 kilograms (70 pounds) of clothing and shoes per year.

Problem is, when we see facts like these, or hear a speech from a climate change scientist, or a professor, or a doctor or researcher, we're

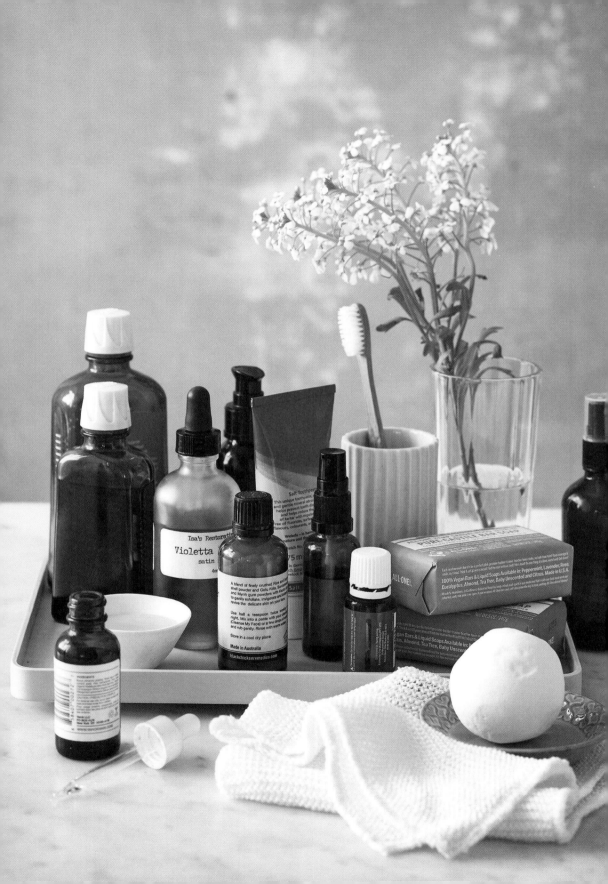

often left feeling despair. We ask ourselves: 'How on earth do I join the dots of these humongous global challenges in health and the environment and do anything big enough to make a difference and affect the outcome?'

THE GOOD NEWS

• • • • • •

I believe that big shifts can result from the simple micro-actions of millions of people coming together.

We can't keep waiting for great news in the headlines. It'll never come if we just continue on. It's up to us to *be* the great news. It's people like you and me, making changes as we go about our day-to-day lives, who incite curiosity from friends. From there, we answer their questions. From there, they make some changes. From there, someone alters the canteen menu, starts buying recycled-textile business cards, ditches the synthetic food colourings or processed foods, gives a community talk, tosses out the synthetic air fresheners at the gym they own ... and on and on we go, until huge multinationals actually take genetically modified sugar beets out of iconic chocolate brands like Hershey's and tinned soups like Campbell's, synthetic colourings out of some of the biggest names in confectionery, setting 100 per cent sustainability goals as IKEA has done, organising $150 million task forces to move away from petroleum-based plastics as LEGO has, or promising to detail the ingredients under the umbrella term 'fragrance' as Unilever has ...

They're not going to make what we're not going to buy, and after working in grassroots education in this area for the past six years I know this: we're the instigators of this change because we've started waking up. And once we're awake, we're not comfortable buying much of the stuff we used to buy every day, eyes wide shut. Once we're not buying it, they've either got to change or go bust. I can picture them in their shareholder meetings, looking at consumer-trend graphs, seeing the big spike in greener options, and knowing that with steady growth in that trend, it's now beyond a trend. It's what more and more of us want, and so they know *they* need to change, however challenging that might be for them, if they want to stay in business. A shift is coming, led by you and me. So don't go saying you're powerless against huge global issues, because if we do it together as millions of people, it becomes a barefoot walk in the park with the soft, pesticide-free grass between our toes.

I believe that big shifts can result from the simple micro-actions of millions of people coming together.

THE NEW FACE OF ACTIVISM

• • • • • •

You. Yes, that's right. For too long, matters of health and the environment have been politicised. For too long, activism has been portrayed as something 'crazy' people do – those greenie 'lunatics'. We see pictures in the media of death-defying acts like swinging off boats, and we don't – and perhaps can't – relate. But now, fully awake, realising our personal power and with reinvigorated critical thinking skills, we can be peaceful, powerful activists in our everyday lives.

DISCOVERY, NOT DEPRIVATION

A key component of successful change is entering into it with a mindset of discovery rather than deprivation. In the discovery of all that is good and true, let the old fall away. There's no deprivation here. We're redefining quality and what's desirable.

Be grateful for this opportunity to fine-tune in this area, make discoveries and explore alternatives. It's not negative. It's not stressful. It's our privilege to do this. However you do it, and however long it takes, is fine. The point is you've started and that you're going to continue. I still today, after starting a decade ago, have big-ticket things I'm working towards. Am I stressed? No. I'm doing my best for today, for now, for my budget. Comfort in feeling that it's enough until the next day, when I can do a little better again, discovering a new idea or resource or motivation.

> *However you do it, and however long it takes, is fine. The point is you've started.*

Whatever your current budget or frame of mind allows *is enough*. It's a journey of a good year or two with little continuing tweaks, and then a decade or more for the bigger-picture stuff. So I offer up this little thought to those who need it:

> BE PROUD OF THAT LITTLE CHANGE YOU'RE
> GOING TO MAKE TODAY. BE PROUD OF THE PLANS
> YOU'RE LAYING OUT AS TIME, CIRCUMSTANCE
> AND ENERGY PERMIT.

If you do the work to truly understand how something doesn't serve us, it will fall off your tree and it will feel quite natural that it goes. Then, if you find a way to incorporate the new 'thing' in a way that doesn't set you back financially, and performs as well or tastes as good, if not better, then it's a no-brainer. That's where this book will come in rather handy for you!

Understand what's what, ditch the stuff that doesn't serve you or the planet, and find simple, gorgeous, delicious new ways to do things, whatever your budget or time constraints. I hope that it will become beautifully obvious to you what needs to be done, that you'll *want* to do it, and then go off on your low tox way with the priorities and time frame that work for you.

MIND THE 'GREENWASHING'

The words 'organic' and 'natural' can be used on food and cosmetics labels, but without certification they mean very little, and the products can still contain dubious ingredients. Over time, once you know your ingredients, you'll start to see the fake green unravelling before your eyes. Don't be disheartened if you get – or have been – caught out here and there as you become better at ingredient-reading.

You'll see pictures of the earth or mothers holding babies in a field full of dandelions advertising products with ingredients known to disrupt our hormones. You'll see slogans like 'Fresh Air System' only to discover that the best form of fresh air is the free form, where you open a window rather than pump synthetic fragrances through your home. You'll see '100 per cent cotton', only to discover that your fellow human was paid peanuts to produce that garment and the dyes are toxic. You'll see 'Made with real fruit' only to find that, in addition to the 5 per cent real fruit, there are 15 other ingredients in there that are anything but real fruit.

Don't be discouraged. It's part of the learning process and developing the skills to know what's what. And it's a beautiful big learning journey ahead.

Once you become aware, what's *not* good and true will start to stand out like a koala on the Eiffel Tower!

Beginners will want to ensure two things:

1 You don't fall into the trap of seeing a few front-of-label ticks saying a product is such-and-such-'free' and assume it's awesome. Whether it's food, cleaning or personal products, those few ticks and catchphrases are on the front in the hope that you're too busy to read the ingredients list, and you just grab it, thinking you're making a great choice.

2 You start to ask these two simple questions: 'How is that made?' and 'Where does that come from?' Yummy caramel crème brûlée tea, eh? *How* exactly do they create that flavour? It can be so super unsettling how many answers you *don't* get that in the end, you'll be running for the eco shops, farmers' market and small providores to take comfort in simple, delicious and transparent truth.

Speaking of the truth, a word on inconvenience ...

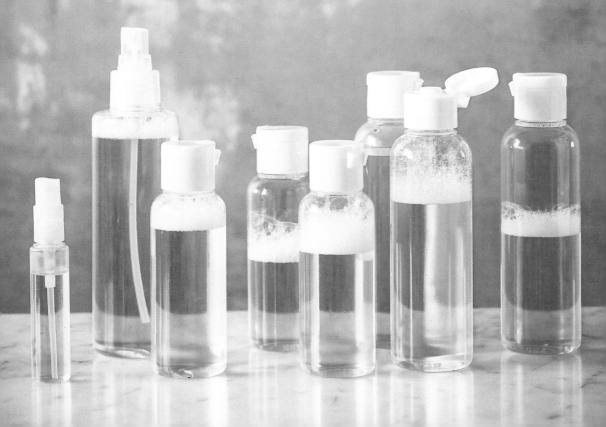

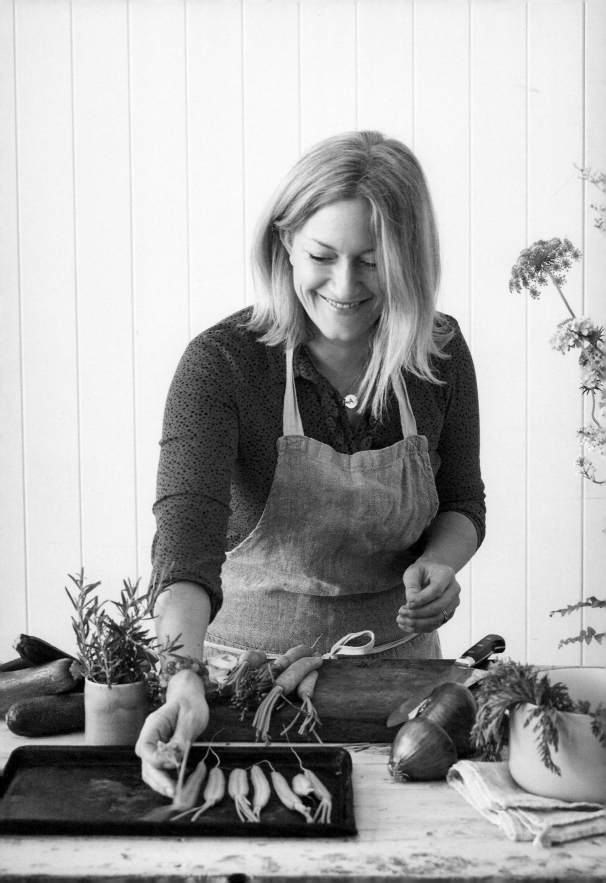

THE INCONVENIENT TRUTH ABOUT CONVENIENCE

They got us so busy that we needed more convenient, time-saving solutions. When we started being sold things like cake mixes, TV dinners and extra-strength washing powder, we were excited rather than dubious, grateful rather than concerned. How nice of them, right, to save us time like that. We got so caught up in their packets and promises that we forgot a quick dinner could be a six-minute steak with fresh vegetables of the season sautéed in butter and herbs. And instead, because they'd defined for us what convenience was, we believed it meant finding a parking space, walking two blocks back up to the takeaway shop, taking a number and standing in a queue until we got to place our order, getting the food all wrapped in plastic, returning to the car and going home ... Sound familiar? They got us goooood!

Take a look at this convenience item – packaged as a time-saver – I once found in the supermarket. It's 125 grams (4½ oz) of chicken breast (with a few bonus, suspect additives), sliced and ready to go as a salad topper, or in a sandwich or stir-fry. I laughed at the 'handy resealable pouch' claim. It's supposedly 2.5 serves – I guess that's to get you needing to snack all afternoon on more convenience foods and thus spend more money, because 50 grams (1¾ oz) of chicken sure ain't much – unless you're a three-year-old.

For 125 grams of non-organic chicken, I worked out that it was nearly three times the price per kilo of buying whole organic, pasture-raised chicken. There's zero cost convenience at all when you compare the price per kilo, and I've since observed similar examples elsewhere. Heck, a tinned processed ham 'meat' is more expensive per kilo than organic chicken. *Que?* So while it might seem like a good, cheap single-serve lunch option with a couple of crackers and tomato, it turns out to be quite expensive compared to what you could have prepared with nothing but the leftovers from a simple meal the night before. Roast two chooks (Australian for 'chickens') at once. Eat one with the family on the night, turning the leftovers into a soup with vegies the next. Cut up the other chicken and freeze it for future grab-and-go meals. Use all the bones for stock - free stock - that can bubble away with some vegetable offcuts while you relax, read or catch up on your favourite show. *That's* convenience.

So, with a simple big-picture-thinking exercise, we saved on the additives, we ensured the ethics of the farming practices, we saved on the price, the plastics volume and the synthetic salt, and instead we defined *real* convenience and saving, whether it's time or money. And we've sent a powerful ripple out about the kind of world we want to fund.

Our ability to make a difference to our health and the health of the planet lies in our every food and home decision. We are in control of our dollars and we *can* make a difference.

The price of so-called convenience is always paid somewhere else down the line. And often, as it turns out, that product is no more convenient than the low tox alternative.

DON'T PANIC!

• • • • • •

When you lift the lid on 'convenience' for the first time as you go through this book and think about your home and your food, it's common to feel a flood of emotions – guilt, anger, confusion, embarrassment, panic. 'How did I not know?' you'll ask yourself. 'How did I not wonder? What would things be like if ... What am I going to do without ...?'

Here's the shift: we don't *part* with convenience on this journey, we just redefine it. Slowly. Conventional messages about convenience lose their appeal pretty quickly. You'll seek a new form of convenience that aligns with your values this time, because you've slowed down enough to define your values. How sweet is that? Truth and peace of mind, coupled with smart buying and smart 'making', become far more important over the course of this journey. Through empowered choice, we know for a fact that we're now on the trajectory of doing the best we can for both our health and the planet's. And we've found a way to make it simple and uncomplicated ... Well bingo, that's our convenience born again – this time, though, as the love child of hippie parents.

So now let's take a look at the major nasties – and low tox alternatives – for our face, body, home and food; discover delicious recipes; and check in with our low tox state of mind for dessert. Sound like a plan?

Oh, and one last thing ... it would be irresponsible of me to not to remind you – and us all, really – that research is constantly evolving, and while I'm sharing everything I've discovered that doesn't sit right with me after my own quest for answers, I invite you wholeheartedly to do your own due diligence and come to your own conclusions.

CHAPTER TWO

·······

LOW TOX
BODY

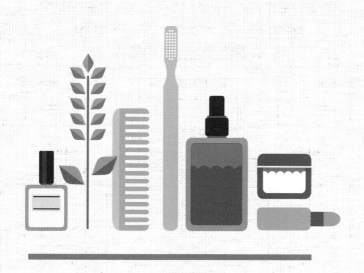

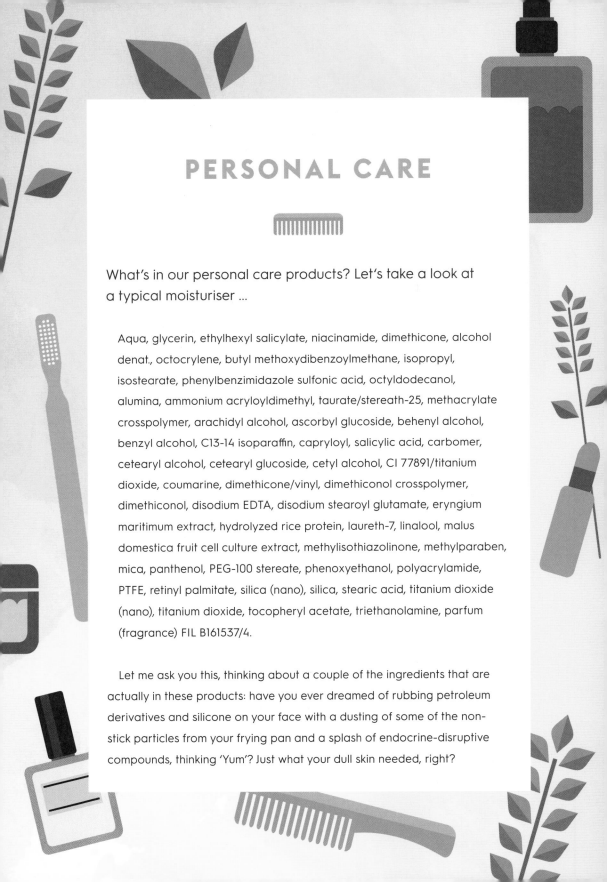

PERSONAL CARE

What's in our personal care products? Let's take a look at a typical moisturiser …

Aqua, glycerin, ethylhexyl salicylate, niacinamide, dimethicone, alcohol denat., octocrylene, butyl methoxydibenzoylmethane, isopropyl, isostearate, phenylbenzimidazole sulfonic acid, octyldodecanol, alumina, ammonium acryloyldimethyl, taurate/stereath-25, methacrylate crosspolymer, arachidyl alcohol, ascorbyl glucoside, behenyl alcohol, benzyl alcohol, C13-14 isoparaffin, capryloyl, salicylic acid, carbomer, cetearyl alcohol, cetearyl glucoside, cetyl alcohol, CI 77891/titanium dioxide, coumarine, dimethicone/vinyl, dimethiconol crosspolymer, dimethiconol, disodium EDTA, disodium stearoyl glutamate, eryngium maritimum extract, hydrolyzed rice protein, laureth-7, linalool, malus domestica fruit cell culture extract, methylisothiazolinone, methylparaben, mica, panthenol, PEG-100 stereate, phenoxyethanol, polyacrylamide, PTFE, retinyl palmitate, silica (nano), silica, stearic acid, titanium dioxide (nano), titanium dioxide, tocopheryl acetate, triethanolamine, parfum (fragrance) FIL B161537/4.

Let me ask you this, thinking about a couple of the ingredients that are actually in these products: have you ever dreamed of rubbing petroleum derivatives and silicone on your face with a dusting of some of the non-stick particles from your frying pan and a splash of endocrine-disruptive compounds, thinking 'Yum'? Just what your dull skin needed, right?

Of course! Or have you ever just picked up a few tiny plastic balls and rubbed them into your leg and thought: 'Mmmmm, just what I needed to feel refreshed and exfoliated, and help my skin feel alive'? Or have you ever thought, 'I'm going to choose that one, because with more phthalates in it, hopefully my partner's sperm count will decrease right in time for us to try for a baby'?

Thought not.

So why, when disguised in pretty pots and tubes like the product opposite, with a picture of an 18-year-old model promising us that our 40-year-old skin can look like theirs, do we buy this stuff? How do we not see it for what it truly is? You and I, potentially responsible for big budgets at work, whole companies or divisions, running a restaurant or an accounting firm, responsible for the safety of our children throughout the day, making analytical decision after analytical decision – and yet never once analysing what we put on our faces and bodies? Are you as perplexed as I am by that? That we could get through 13 years of school, then college and/or university and never wonder what was in everything we used each day.

Now ... Equally important is not to panic about everything you don't understand the chemical name for. Is it all bad? Absolutely not. You often hear, 'You want to get all those chemicals out,' but this is misleading. We ourselves are chemicals. Water is a chemical substance. Peppermint oil is made up of multiple chemicals. The humble blueberry contains well more than 20 chemical compounds. There's no room for fear-mongering nor unfounded alarmism here. Many chemicals have been researched extensively and are harmless. Are some of them sufficiently dubious to have us exercise caution? Yes, yes, they are. Should we learn more about what's in our products? Yes, we absolutely should, and in this section we're going to get to know those main nasties, because once you know those, you'll be able to spot them and know straight away not to continue considering that product. We'll also look at some simple, delicious alternatives. And to carry on the learning, you can head to lowtoxlife.com/book-resources.

THE TOP SKINCARE NASTIES: ENDOCRINE DISRUPTORS

• • • •

It's essential to understand what we're leaving behind, and it will ultimately add to your excitement and sense of accomplishment when you make the switch to simpler alternatives. I promise!

The endocrine system is made up of several glands that produce hormones. Endocrine disruptors can mimic or partly mimic our naturally occurring hormones. They can also bind to a hormone receptor within a cell and stop the natural hormone from binding. And they can block or interfere with the way our hormones are controlled. Any woman knows that it's hard enough to balance your hormones on the best of days, without a whole bunch of little hormone-mimicking, -binding or -blocking missiles firing around in your body.

Endocrine disruptors affect multiple systems in the body and contribute to lowered sperm counts, precocious puberty, endometriosis, PCOS, thyroid dysregulation, testicular cancer and breast cancer. More recently, they've been shown to play a role in metabolic dysfunction and obesity,

PRO TIP

Download the Chemical Maze App or the Environmental Working Group's (EWG) Skin Deep App if you're unsure about other ingredients. For me, though, seeing any of the main nasties listed in this section means I don't have to continue trying to decipher the other ingredients. It's a no.

leading biologist Bruce Blumberg of the University of California, Irvine to coin the term 'obesogen' in 2006. This was originally pooh-poohed by the scientific community, but with more and more mounting evidence and trials, he's now heralded as a pioneer. In 2009 the Endocrine Society, an 86-year-old medical association, published the first paper in its history detailing the link between these chemicals and increases in disease. When one of America's oldest medical societies says 'these links can no longer be ignored' and calls for new policies to reduce these endocrine-disruptive chemicals, it really is high time for us to sit up and take notice – and action.

There are many endocrine disruptors, but these are the most common you'll find in personal care.

PHTHALATES

These are 'plasticiser compounds' used to make fragrances last longer and certain plastics uber-bendy, soft or stretchy (think of those kids' goopy coloured gels and 'monster slime' from a toyshop, a cheap puzzle play mat, a PVC raincoat, plastic book coverings or vinyl flooring). The good news about phthalates is that we tend to rid our bodies of them quite quickly, unlike some chemicals, which can accumulate in fat tissue and be difficult to get out. Ditching the 'fake smells' from your home is just about the quickest change you can make and detox you can experience. The damage from phthalates is caused by daily, repeated exposure – more than our bodies can handle. The available research studies show that this damage can mean everything from low sperm counts, to asthma, changes in male babies' testes and penis size, increased incidence of breast cancer and tumours.

Ditching the 'fake smells' from your home is just about the quickest change you can make and detox you can experience.

How does a phthalate show up on a label in personal care? Most often under the words 'fragrance' or 'parfum'. A simple thing to do is ask yourself, when you start to analyse the smells in your products, 'Could you naturally make something smell like that from plants?' Unless it has an asterisk and below says 'essential oils', you're dealing with a synthetic fragrance, and in the vast majority of products that use synthetic fragrances, the plasticiser is almost always there to ensure the scent stays for days. If you're unsure, email the company that makes the product.

PARABENS

Parabens can mimic oestrogen. They've been detected in human breast cancer tissues, suggesting a possible association between parabens in cosmetics and cancer, although studies haven't been conclusive. Parabens may also interfere with male reproductive functions. It will be named on the ingredients list, so it's an easy one.

PHENOXYETHANOL

Some studies say this is safe in low concentrations, but they admit this isn't taking into account other uses and synergistic effects if there are other endocrine disruptors in the product. The Dow Chemical safety data sheet for this chemical cites animal studies where repeated exposure affected the red blood cells, kidney, liver, thyroid gland and respiratory tract. It's up to you where you draw the line, but when there's doubt and the studies call for more research, it makes sense to me to exercise caution and avoid this.

RESOURCINOL

A hormone disruptor found in hair dyes and used in face and body products to break down tough, scaly skin.

BENZOPHINONE

A possible hormone disruptor (evidence found in animal trials) used to protect things from UV light and found in some sunscreens, lipsticks and nail polishes, as well as sunglasses and food packaging.

TRIPHENYL PHOSPHATE

An endocrine disruptor used mostly in nail polishes. Research shows that constant exposure can lead to reproductive changes and weight gain.

OTHER NASTIES

Now onto other nasties that regularly feature in body-care products:

* **Sodium lauryl sulfate, sodium laureth sulfate:** The former is fine in cleaning products provided it's not derived from petroleum or unsustainable palm oil, but neither is acceptable for personal care. Skin irritants both, and the latter is also a suspected carcinogen. Seeing '-eth' in an ingredient is a clue that it could be contaminated with 1,4-dioxane, deemed by the EPA a likely carcinogen based on extensive animal studies.

* **Triclosan:** Found in antibacterial products, especially hand washes and acne-targeting face washes. Damaging to the thyroid gland and good bacteria, it was banned by the US Food and Drug Administration (FDA) in November 2016, with a phase-out plan by 2018. This is not a global ban, so it's important to keep it on your radar.

* **PEGs:** These petroleum-based polymer derivatives (PEG is the abbreviation of polyethylene glycol) are used in cosmetics as emollients (to soften the skin)s and emulsifiers (which facilitate the mixing of oil- and water-based ingredients).

* **Benzoic acid, sodium benzoate:** These are a common cause of eczema, dermatitis, psoriasis and hives. Avoid them unless the label states that they're naturally derived.

* **Polyquaternium 7:** It's a synthetic quaternary ammonium compound, and a known eye irritant.

- ❋ **Methylisothiazolinone:** This is one of the most popular preservatives since consumers turned against parabens. It has caused a marked rise in skin irritations, namely contact dermatitis.
- ❋ **Carbomer/polymers:** A carbomer is any series of polymers of acrylic acid used to thicken and smooth cosmetics. Mmm, acrylics on my face.
- ❋ **Benzaldehyde, benzocaine, benzophenone, benzyl alcohol:** These similar chemicals have been shown to cause skin irritability (such as contact dermatitis).
- ❋ **Butoxyethanol:** This member of the glycol ether family is a butyl ether of ethylene glycol, which is used as a car coolant … Hmmm, on my face?
- ❋ **Ceteareth/ceteareth-20:** This is particularly dodgy if used on damaged, sensitive skin. EWG has found it to contain the carcinogen 1,4-dioxane.
- ❋ **Microbeads:** These are touted for their 'active' scouring and exfoliating properties, but the real story behind them is plastic. Plastic that often contains phthalates and BPA. There can be as many as 350,000 plastic beads in a single tube, floating over your face – some perhaps even accidentally into your mouth (or not so accidentally when they're found in toothpastes! It's okay, you can laugh, cry, laugh now. Totally acceptable!) – and then out through the drain, into the waterways, into the fish, then back out of the sea, lightly steamed with ginger and shallots and onto our dinner plates. No thanks. They make zero sense.

If you're starting to feel a sense of rage that it's considered perfectly fine for this stuff to be present in droves in our mainstream body and face products, then welcome to the club. I felt a huge sense of injustice and disbelief when starting to read the research on so many ingredients in personal care. Feel that anger but don't misdirect it towards yourself or your parents. We didn't know. It's not our fault. We do know now, however, so use that knowledge as the fire in your belly to make beautiful changes. Whether you take the DIY route or buy low tox brands, you can check out the guide at lowtoxlife.com/book-resources.

THERE IS AN ALTERNATIVE

The good news, when it comes to natural beauty, is that we can do so much to enhance our gorgeous natural gifts! Yes, I said gifts. It's time we stopped letting mega-brands make us feel like we're never beautiful enough. Imagine if we put all the energy we waste on thinking we're not enough into outward kindness and meaningful work! Besides, a lot of the common skin complaints can mean we're missing something nutritionally or we could do with a natural boost or lifestyle tweak.

And an admission: I'm not a huge skincare product DIYer. I make a few things that I love and that you'll see in the following pages, but DIY isn't a priority for me. I make my serums and my scrubs and my delicious body lotion bars as well as a token face mask every now and then, but I actually love supporting low tox brands and businesses, and saving myself the time, so I'm comfortable with a mix of both bought and homemade. If you want to go all in on the DIY, great. The recipes in this book are divine. If you want to buy your essentials and prioritise time differently, that's totally fine. Remember, change doesn't stick if we do it someone else's way, so have a play, have a shop around and come up with a personal care plan that's going to work for you!

FACE CARE

I started out my professional life in cosmetics at Downtown Duty Free in Sydney's Strand Arcade. I then went on to work for two luxury cosmetics brands.

In our staff training sessions, we'd always talk about the rare algae of the so-and-so sea, or the organic extracted collagen or the pure vitamin C or the fact that the formula could penetrate below the epidermis to the dermis or that the formula was non comedogenic (wouldn't clog the pores). We always talked about the 'top half' of the ingredients, the 'actives', the 'features', the 'performance'. Never once was the bottom half of the label addressed, where all the nasties typically lie.

Over the years, I met so many women in the industry. On the cosmetics floor it seemed that all of us had a hormonal issue. It was the topic of endless conversation and confusion on a quiet Tuesday morning. Endometriosis, polycystic ovarian syndrome (PCOS), fertility issues, super-painful periods ... I'd never heard of such things until then. When I was 22, however, I was diagnosed with PCOS myself. Whether or not this was related, I'll never know, but continually emerging science seems to suggest that it's a possibility.

So many products were selling a promise of some kind, yet I later realised that these expensive products are often short-lived bandaids for issues far better addressed with lifestyle changes or advice from a health practitioner!

These expensive products are often short-lived bandaids ...

WRINKLES

Your skin will have either deep wrinkles from ageing, sun or lack of healthy fats *or* fine feathery lines from dehydration. You'll go a very long way towards vibrant skin simply by remembering to drink water when you're thirsty, and by including animal fats from pasture-raised animals, fish oil, linseeds (flaxseeds), quality dairy, avocado, coconut oil and nuts in your daily foods. It doesn't 'cost' you, this beauty tactic, simply because you'd be eating anyway, so it's just about tweaking what you're already doing so you can feed your skin from the inside.

SAG

Are you saying bye-bye to more collagen and elastin than you'd care to? Simple DIY facial oil blends boosted with essential oils can be a godsend here. Copaiba, neroli, frankincense, carrot seed and lemon essential oils are all excellent support in this department. I have two little amber-glass pump bottles, one for am, one for pm (see page 48).

DULLNESS

Try using plain honey as your cleanser, and for an extra boost of brightness, add a drop of geranium essential oil. Works a treat if you combine this daily morning practice with a weekly skin polish/exfoliation and good hydration on the inside and out.

DARK CIRCLES

Dark circles need you to get to the root cause, and the answer isn't in the bottom of your next pot of eye cream! According to some sources, the three most common things they can mean are food intolerances, mouth-breathing when you sleep (instead of breathing through your nose with your mouth shut) and liver congestion. Best you talk to a qualified practitioner for your individual assessment if you're a 'dark circles' person.

MY MORNING AND EVENING ESSENTIAL OIL SERUMS

My morning oil is copaiba, neroli and frankincense (a.k.a 'franky') – 3 drops of each in 30 ml (1 fl oz) of carrier oil (I use rosehip oil) in an amber glass dropper bottle. I use a few drops of this mixture each morning before my moisturiser. Copaiba and frankincense are perfect for the morning 'de-puff', and neroli doubles as a mood-lifter.

For the evening, I do lemon and carrot seed oils together (I don't use lemon in the day as it's photosensitive), then add vetiver oil – 3 drops of each in 30 ml (1 fl oz) of carrier oil, and all in an amber dropper bottle. Vetiver is an earthy sleep precursor that's been shown to support skin tone. Let it all do the hard yards while you sleep. Use this serum alone, or with a night cream for further antioxidants and hydration, especially if you have fine, feathery dehydration lines.

PUFFINESS

It's laughable the amount of money I used to convince people to spend on de-puffing their eyes. Here are three cheap and safe remedies for puffiness:

1. Get more sleep. It does so much for us and we could all do with more, preferably starting by 11 pm so we get some good hormone-regenerative 'golden time'.

2. Lie down for 5 minutes with a cucumber slice on each eye. They really do magically de-puff, and the forced slow-down is beautiful too.

3 Rinse your face in the morning with very cold water or, better still, take a fully cold shower after your hot one, just for 30 seconds if you can work up to that. You'll drastically speed up your 'I've been awake for ages' look. Then use the morning serum opposite. *What* puff? There is none!

ACNE

So often, people with acne are given the most toxic stuff going. It frequently has high levels of triclosan, for its unproven antibacterial effects, as well as microbeads, sodium lauryl/laureth sulfate and more. Prescription medication can also cause other nasty side effects. You could try these ways instead:

* Work with a health practitioner to see if any hormone imbalances, nutrient deficiencies or lifestyle issues might be at play. Treating topically is a bandaid solution when often a root cause needs to be uncovered.
* Grab yourself a bottle of a high-quality tea-tree/melaleuca essential oil and apply 1–3 drops with 3 drops jojoba oil, straight onto the acne areas for its antibacterial and anti-inflammatory properties.
* Make yourself a facial night-time oil in a pump or glass dropper bottle, with 1 tablespoon jojoba oil and 2 teaspoons castor oil, which has anti-inflammatory properties and is great for oily skin. Jojoba is similar to the oil in our sebum and can send the message to our oil production 'factory' to slow down producing so much oil itself. Then add 10 drops melaleuca oil, 5 drops rosemary oil, 5 drops lavender oil, 5 drops clary sage and 5 drops eucalyptus oil. Before bed, apply a small pump of this to the acne-prone areas on your body, avoiding the eye area.
* Use a very mild cleansing milk to wash, rather than a harsh foam that strips the skin and in the long run increases sebum production and sets you on a vicious cycle of needing to wash more. No good!
* Mix up a toner of 1 tablespoon steeped and cooled green tea and 1 teaspoon apple cider vinegar, with 5 drops orange essential oil for its astringent properties. Use for 2–3 days then remake.

DIY FACE-CARE ALTERNATIVES

• • • • • •

Here are some basic recipes to get you started, but if you want more, get adventuring online – sites like Pinterest can be a fantastic resource and inspiration. Alternatively, if you're not the DIY kind, or you want to mix and match, check out my country-specific guides and favourite brands and products for all skin types at lowtoxlife.com/book-resources.

THE CHEAPEST, SIMPLEST DIYS

The Low Tox Life is not elitist. There's always something for every budget. Try these incredibly simple face-care options:

* **plain coconut oil** – as an eye make-up remover at the end of the day!
* **honey** – pure, plain, raw honey makes a perfect face cleanser. Rub it onto your face, then rinse off with warm water. Delicious! I know it sounds weird, but just try it!

FACE SCRUB

MAKES 1 application

1 teaspoon coarsely ground tapioca
   pearls or rice (you want the texture
   of polenta; use a good blender)

2 teaspoons honey
1–2 teaspoons hot water, or as
   needed

Mix the ground tapioca into the honey, adding the hot water if the honey is super thick. Massage the scrub into your face, leave for 1 minute then rinse off with warm water for deliciously baby-smooth skin.

FACE MASKS

It's so easy and fun to make your own!

HYDRATING
MAKES 3 masks

1 tablespoon honey

¼ avocado, mashed

2 tablespoons coconut milk kefir

Mix all the ingredients in a small bowl then pass through a sieve and refrigerate for up to 1 week. Apply every 2 days as a boost until used up.

CLARIFYING AND FIRMING
MAKES 1 mask

1 teaspoon bentonite clay

1 teaspoon activated charcoal

3 drops carrot seed oil

3 drops copaiba essential oil

15 ml (1 fl oz) aloe vera gel

Mix carefully (hello charcoal!) in a small bowl. Before your shower, apply to your face and leave on for 10 minutes. Rinse off in the shower.

PURIFYING
MAKES 1 treatment

My friend Cybele Masterman taught me this one, and it's brilliant!

1 strawberry

Eat the bottom half of the fruit, then rub the remaining berry onto your face, avoiding the eye area. Sounds strange, I know, but leave the juices on for 5 minutes so the fruit acids can work their magic, then rinse off.

AMANDA COOK'S HOT CLOTH CLEANSER

MAKES about 80 ml (2½ fl oz)

My friend Amanda, a DIY talent, taught me this, and I'm thoroughly addicted. Each jar of cleanser should last for a year – if you don't use it all up first!

Pro tip: When working with beeswax, keep a designated DIY toolset just for recipes that include it, as it's a nightmare to remove completely from utensils and bowls, and can clog up sinks easily. Keep a spoon, a stainless-steel bowl for your double boiler/bain-marie and a grater in a bag with your block of beeswax, and you won't need to clean them after use.

25 g (1 oz) castor oil

25 g (1 oz) olive oil

30 g (1 oz) cocoa butter, or shea
   butter for those with clogged pores

20 g (¾ oz) beeswax

7 drops rosemary essential oil

7 drops eucalyptus essential oil

6 drops lavender essential oil

Weigh the castor oil, olive oil, cocoa butter and beeswax into a heatproof bowl. In a bain-marie or double boiler (the heatproof bowl over a saucepan of boiling water), stir until the beeswax and cocoa butter are melted.

Remove from the heat and stir in the oils. Pour into jars and allow to cool, then close with a lid, and label with the product name, ingredients and date.

To use, scoop out some cleanser with a fingertip. Rub it between your fingers and then onto your face to melt. Massage it into your skin with circular motions. You might want to massage it in for 2 minutes, concentrating on those areas that need deep cleansing (nose, forehead and chin). Run the tap until the water is hot to the hand, and wet your washcloth thoroughly. Wring out the washcloth, and place the hot cloth over your face for a couple of minutes. If it cools off, just rinse again in hot water and put back on your face. Gently wipe off the cleanser with the hot washcloth. Finish with a splash of cool water. All clean and totally self-loved.

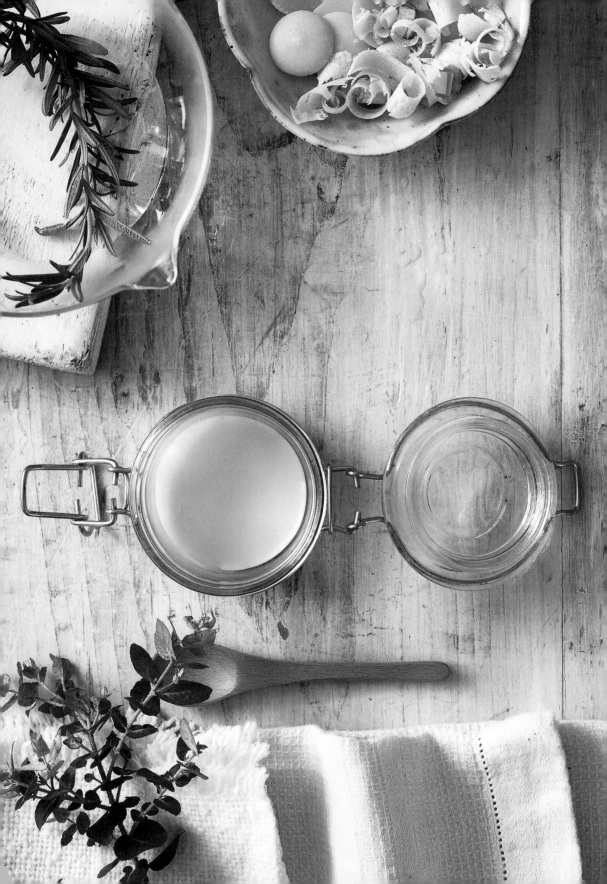

FACE MIST/TONER

Fill a small 30 ml (1 fl oz) pump spray bottle with witch hazel. Add 1 teaspoon vitamin E (I break open 1–2 quality mixed tocopherol capsules for this) and 5 drops rosemary oil – amazingly invigorating at the start of the day.

PRO TIPS FOR SHOPPING ONLINE

• • • • • •

Not a DIYer? Only shop from sites that make their full ingredients lists available readily. If you have to click through to five different pages and request a PDF, chances are there's a reason, in my experience. Nothing to hide equals high trust, and that's what we want.

If you love a product and it seems low tox but you're not sure, become a serial emailer. Most customer service people will reply promptly to your questions, so go for it. Come from a place of kindness, not judgement. They didn't create the formula. They're just a hard-working person with a job to do, so keyboard hating on a customer service rep will only weigh heavily on your heart in the end and achieve nothing.

Finally, repeat this mantra after me: *Simplify, don't complicate*. If anything, this is not about spending *more*, but deciding exactly what you need and buying less, but better, of non-toxic quality and throwing a few simple DIYs into the mix. *And* that doesn't break the bank. All this stuff is much less expensive than prestige cosmetics. Bonus, right?

Simplify, don't complicate.

Discover my favourite brands internationally at lowtoxlife.com/book-resources.

✳ TO DO! ✳

✓ Commit to simplifying your skincare products. Do you really need everything you've been using? You might find that everything needs replacing.

✓ Decide what you're going to toss, what you're going to buy and what you're going to make yourself.

✓ Implement something new when it feels right to – it's not a contest!

Note: When tossing things, be sure to squeeze the rest out into the bin rather than the sink, and then recycle the packaging if you're not going to reuse it. There are some amazing recycling services like TerraCycle, which you can look into. You could also consider donating what you won't use. Some people feel comfortable with this, others feel it's wrong knowing it's not great for you. Your call. There's no right or wrong.

MAKE-UP

Make-up is yet another place where SO. MUCH. STUFF. HIDES. The irony of 'beauty' is that the products in this category exist to make you feel better about yourself, yet they compromise your health in the long term – and the health of future generations and the environment.

There are a few big nasties, apart from the ones already covered on pages 40–44, that commonly appear in make-up.

BIG NASTIES IN MAKE-UP

• • • • • •

I find it's best to know a few 'key' baddies, because if a product is dubious, it will always display at least one or two from my non-negotiable toxin list, so from there you can just walk away … No need to keep reading through the rest of the list – it'd take hours to decipher them all!

Micas, pigments and titanium dioxides are in most make-ups. Some people are sensitive, some aren't, so you'll have to decide what works for you and what doesn't.

TALC

This mineral has inconclusive yet strong links to ovarian cancer, which is thought to correlate with the fact that it can be contaminated with asbestos. Do we want to wait to find out? It's a no from me, as I exercise the precautionary principle! Get it off your baby's bottom and out of your powders and eye shadows.

LEAD

Love that red lippy? Well, it's probably got lead in it. Elevated lead in adults has been found to lead to miscarriages, birth defects and seizures. If you want peace of mind, ask companies for lead-testing reports.

CADMIUM

Lippies again ... you'll often find it there! Cadmium is a carcinogen that has been found in breast cancer biopsies and is thought to cause cancer cells to multiply. All I can say is, how is this allowed in stuff sold to women?!

MUSKS

Used as fragrances, often in pressed and loose powders, these can accumulate in the body, and have been linked in laboratory studies to skin irritation, hormone disruption and cancer.

TOLUENE

Made from petroleum or coal tar, this is found in most synthetic fragrances. Chronic exposure is linked to anaemia, lowered blood cell counts, and liver or kidney damage, and may affect a developing fetus.

MINERAL OIL, PARAFFIN AND PETROLATUM (PETROLEUM JELLY)

While these products can be useful in emergency medical settings for their low skin reactivity and barrier-creating properties, their raw material is petroleum and they can possibly accumulate in our tissues (if we, for example, swallow a lip balm containing them). They also trap heat and don't allow the skin to breathe. They do nothing to nourish our skin, when we could instead be using natural oils and ingredients that do. As a cheeky aside, mineral oil in inks has been found to tamper with our oestrogen levels.

BHA/BHT

Butylated hydroxyanisole and acid butylated hydroxytoluene, used as preservatives in make-up, skincare products and even food, are thought to be endocrine disruptors and protentially to cause asthma and skin irritation.

SILOXANES

These ingredients, which will end in '-siloxane' or '-methicone', are used in a variety of cosmetics to soften, smooth and moisten. They are suspected endocrine disruptors, and cyclotetrasiloxane is thought to be a reproductive toxicant. And they're harmful to fish and other wildlife.

NANOPARTICLES

Often found in SPF face powders, sunscreens and other cosmetics, these can, as the name suggests, be *tiny*, and thus cause concern about inhalation and environmental contamination as they accumulate in the environment over time with as-yet unknown effects Based on this alone, I would use one of the many available nano-free options.

WHAT MAKE-UP CAN WE USE?

• • • • • •

First of all, challenge yourself with the question 'What do I simply *not* need to replace?' Often we realise we just don't need everything we've got, so we probably won't need to replace every little thing. That's the beauty of increasing our awareness of what we buy in the first place.

Toss out what you don't need. Feel the delicious feeling of letting go of 'stuff' that doesn't serve you, like the eye shadow set you got for your 18th that you felt rude not keeping – we've all been there!

To replace what you do decide you want to use regularly and enjoy, there are brands out there that *are* doing the right thing.

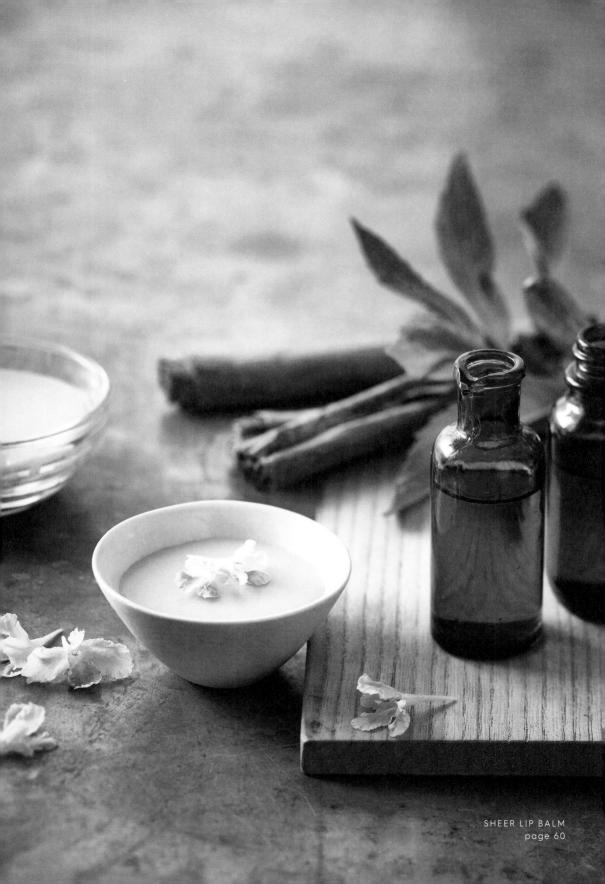

SHEER LIP BALM
page 60

SHEER LIP BALM

MAKES 65 ml (2¼ fl oz)

This is so easy. You can keep back tubes from old lip balms you're finishing up, fill them with this and refrigerate to set. Or, you can buy a little pot and fill it. For some shimmer you could add the face-highlighting powder.

2 tablespoons beeswax pastilles or grated beeswax

2 tablespoons cocoa butter

2 tablespoons coconut oil

5 drops peppermint essential oil

2 drops cinnamon essential oil

1 teaspoon shimmer face-highlighting powder (optional)

Melt the beeswax, cocoa butter and coconut oil in a double boiler (a heatproof bowl over a saucepan of boiling water). Once melted, remove from the heat, add the essential oils and powder (if using), and decant into your chosen containers.

WHAT'S IN MY OWN MAKE-UP BAG?

• • • • • •

These days I have a cheek tint, a mineral foundation for the T-zone, an illuminator to keep me brightened up, a mascara, BB (beauty balm) cream and sheer eye shadow, along with one sheer lippy, one lip gloss and one bright red for 'that night' of the year, along with a few other pieces! Simple, and a far cry from the ginormous three-tiered make-up 'chest' I used to have back in the day ... Although I only used a tenth of it, of course.

Pro tip: Many online green beauty sites offer sample foundations or a colour-matching service. Investigate this, as being able to have a try first can save you time and money. And be patient – the right product is out there.

BODY CARE AND SUNSCREEN

Our skin is our largest organ, and our outer body makes up a large part of our skin's surface, so that's a whole lotta surface area to be soaking up toxins.

For body lotions and scrubs, it's a matter of applying (love a good pun!) what you've learnt, and choosing better. It's all the same nasties for this category, so there's nothing 'new' to learn on that front. Look out for fake fragrances and microbeads in scrubs, as well as triclosan, parabens, phenoxyethanol, PEGs, propylene glycol and sodium lauryl sulfate ... the usual suspects. Probably my favourite DIYs of all are the Body Lotion Cupcakes (page 62) and the scrubs on page 65.

Tip: As you phase things out, perhaps make a little birthday or Christmas wish list for your family to treat you to a few things when that time comes. Asking for something specific means a) no stuff you don't want or need cluttering up your space, and b) relief from them, knowing they don't have to try to think of something and potentially get it wrong, knowing 'She/He's a hippie now. I don't even know if she/he'll approve of that.'

BODY LOTIONS

• • • • • •

If you're buying a body lotion, you already know the worst nasties to avoid. Fractionated coconut oil or olive oil both make inexpensive and completely toxin-free options. You could also add argan, rosehip or avocado oils to the mix, and personalise them with 3 drops per 20 ml (½ fl oz) of grapefruit, geranium, cypress, rosemary or juniper essential oils – or a combination depending on your preference. All of these oils are brilliant for boosting circulation and supporting even skin texture on the body.

My body lotion cupcakes – yes, you heard me right! – are gorgeous to make for yourself or as gifts, and take no time at all.

BODY LOTION CUPCAKES

MAKES 3–4 large bars

You'll also need some silicone moulds in your preferred shape or paper cupcake liners.

30 g (1 oz/½ cup) grated beeswax
65 g (2¼ oz/½ cup) cocoa butter
125 ml (4 fl oz/½ cup) coconut oil
 (refined for no coconut scent)

25 drops essential oils of your choice
 (e.g. rosemary, vetiver and jasmine,
 or a woody or floral combo)

Melt the beeswax over low heat in a bain-marie or double boiler (a heatproof bowl over a saucepan of boiling water). Once the wax is melted, still over the heat, melt in the cocoa butter. Once the cocoa butter is melted, melt in the coconut oil, stirring well. Remove from the heat and stir in the essential oils. Pour the mixture into your chosen moulds. Wait patiently for them to harden – this will take about 1 hour at room temperature, or you could hurry things along in the fridge.

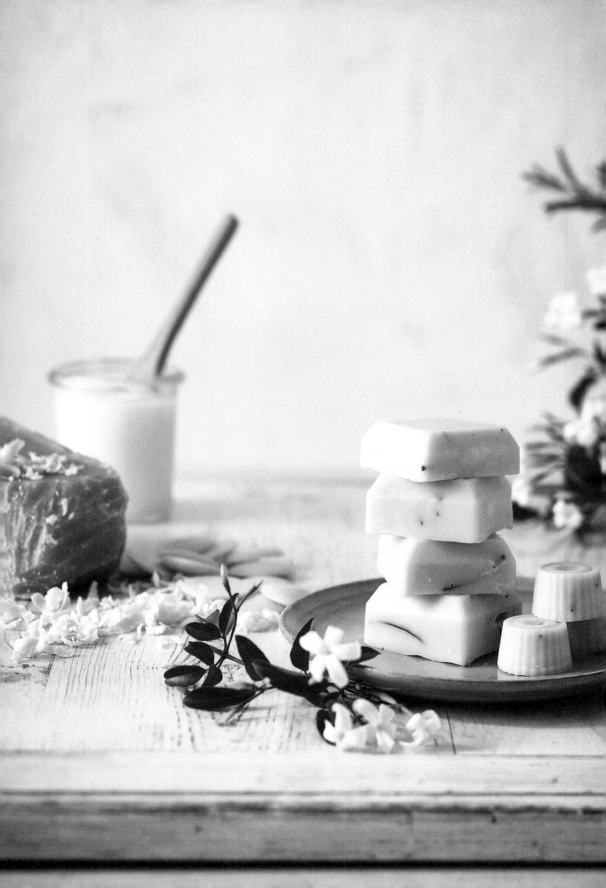

HAND AND BODY SOAPS

· · · · · ·

We've already met most of the nasties in these, but there are a couple more you should look out for.

ANTIBACTERIAL PRODUCTS

We're anti-germ obsessed, yet research suggests that the antibacterial products we've been using in the past couple of decades can lead to antibiotic resistance and potentially allergies in children. Look out for:

* **benzalkonium chloride:** This is a known irritant, reported to cause asthma, dermatitis, eye and skin irritation, and nervous system issues. What's it also in? Asthma inhalers! The world has gone mad.
* **triclosan:** We already know this petroleum-derived chemical can cause thyroid imbalances, but it can also cause skin, eye and lung irritation, and immune system dysfunction, and it can off-gas chloroform when mixed with liquids. It's also an environmental toxin. Great!

SIMPLE DIY HAND AND BODY SOAPS

If you'd like to make your own hand soap, save an old foaming soap dispenser or invest in a beautiful new one. Fill your dispenser with one part Castile soap and three to five parts water, 2 teaspoons olive oil and 10 drops essential oils of your choice. You'll save so much money per litre, it's crazy.

You can't beat a good bar soap or Castile soap for washing the body. Bar soap is also perfect for avoiding plastic wrappings.

BODY SCRUBS

Here are two quick and delicious DIY body scrubs. They make perfect DIY gifts if you want to give from the heart for birthdays or Christmas.

COCONUT, CARAMEL AND LEMON BODY SCRUB

MAKES about 300 ml (10½ fl oz)

A homemade scrub is cheaper and doesn't pollute our oceans or our bodies. And it smells like you could eat it – because in fact you could!

100 ml (3½ fl oz) melted coconut oil or sweet almond oil

105 g (3¾ oz/¾ cup) coconut sugar or organic brown sugar

35 g (1 oz/¼ cup) coarse sea salt (or fine sea salt for your face)

1 tablespoon lemon juice

1 teaspoon grated lemon zest

2 teaspoons vanilla extract (optional)

5 drops rosemary essential oil (optional)

Mix all the ingredients in a medium bowl. Pop in a jar. Stick a ribbon on it. Give it to someone. No, keep it.

COFFEE BODY SCRUB

MAKES enough for 3 uses

This super-simple scrub takes no time to whip up, using spent coffee grounds, coconut oil, sea salt and vanilla extract. It smells divine and is really invigorating.

2 tablespoons coffee grounds

1 tablespoon Celtic Sea, Himalayan or Dead Sea salt, or fleur de sel

2–3 tablespoons coconut oil (see note)

2 teaspoons vanilla bean extract

Mix all the ingredients in a small bowl. Transfer to a jar. That's it.

Note: More oil means a gentler scrub.

SUNSCREENS

• • • • • •

Now it has to be said that I live in a country where sunscreen is non-negotiable. Australian sun is harsher than any other, kind of like our crocs, snakes and spiders – I've been dying to get some Australian stereotyping out of the way, so there it is! That said, it doesn't mean we shouldn't think about what type of sunscreen we're going to use, and as with all categories of products, there are safer options, and dubious ones containing ingredients such as these:

* **octyl methoxycinnamate (OMC):** This is one of the most frequently used chemical UV filters worldwide. OMC easily penetrates the upper layer of the skin and, when exposed to UV radiation, generates damaging free radicals in skin cells.
* **oxybenzone (benzophenone-3), octyl-dimethyl-PABA and octinoxate:** These are all hormone disruptors.
* **4-methylbenzylidene camphor (4-MBC):** Male rats born to mothers exposed to 4-MBC had lower testis weight, and experienced delayed puberty and decreased adult prostate weight. Human trials found that both OMC and 4-MBC were readily absorbed through the skin and were detectable in urine.
* **padimate O (2-ethylhexyl-4-dimethylaminobenzoate):** When exposed to sunlight, this generates free radicals that can cause breaks in DNA strands.

Eek! We're spoilt for choice now, though, in natural and effective sunscreen-land, so watch out for the key nasties to avoid and find a gorgeous local natural one to try – or even brave one of the DIY recipes out there!

There are brilliant low tox sunscreens available these days. Hop over to lowtoxlife.com/book-resources for a starting list.

SELF-TANNING

• • • • • •

If you don't want to get in the sun but you want a glow or you're pale-skinned and want to go a couple of shades darker in the summer time, you might like a little helping hand in the tan and glow department. Problem is, those are often an absolute shocker when it comes to fragrances and other chemicals. Check for the nasties I've listed already when you're shopping. For a natural pigment boost, add a couple of drops of carrot seed oil to the Coffee Body Scrub (page 65) and use it twice weekly.

DEODORANT

• • • • • •

Apart from our old friends the parabens, triclosan and talc, deodorants have their own set of top nasties, but there is good news – although some of you might fear that you'll be smelly, natural deodorant actually does work. You just have to find the one that works for you – it's no different from when you tried a few before settling in with the mainstream one you've been using until now.

ALUMINIUM

Aluminium is the element that makes an antiperspirant do what it says. The way it works as an antiperspirant? Essentially, the aluminium salts block the sweat ducts and prevent you getting sweaty under there. The sweat doesn't stop being produced under the surface, it just doesn't get to the surface. Does that freak anyone else out, given we're meant to sweat as a form of detoxification and body temperature regulation?

TEA & DEA

Triethanolamine and diethanolamine are used here as emulsifiers. They could both be toxic if absorbed into the body over a long period; DEA can cause liver and kidney damage, and TEA allergic reactions. They are already restricted in Europe due to carcinogenic effects, and are worthy of caution.

FD&C COLOURS

Some of these synthetic colours are made from coal-tar derivatives and are known to be carcinogenic; they also often cause allergic skin reactions.

SAFE DIY DEODORANT ALTERNATIVES

Many people swear by these basic DIY options:

* Wipe a slice of citrus under the arm – plain and simple.
* Mix 1 teaspoon aluminium-free bicarbonate of soda (baking soda) with 5 teaspoons arrowroot flour, tapioca flour or organic, non-GMO cornflour (cornstarch). Keep in a jar and sprinkle a little under your arms after your shower. To scent it, add 5 drops rosemary essential oil.
* Coconut oil. This doesn't work for me, but many swear by it.

AMANDA'S LIME AND COCONUT DEODORANT

MAKES about 60 ml (2 fl oz/¼ cup)

This recipe from my talented friend Amanda Cook is so easy!

35 g (1¼ oz/¼ cup) arrowroot or tapioca flour

1 tablespoon bicarbonate of soda (baking soda)

2 tablespoons coconut oil

5 drops lime essential oil or your preferred essential oil

Mix all the ingredients together, transfer to a clean jar or tin and allow to harden before using within 2 months. For easier mixing, melt the coconut oil.

PERIOD CARE

· · · · · ·

We're thought, on average, to use 12,000 tampons over a lifetime, but
don't feel bad if you've never wondered until now what exactly might be
in tampons or pads. Because of their cotton content, they can contain
pesticide residues, synthetic fibres such as rayon, and other chemicals such
as chlorine. Just get excited that today you can start avoiding nasties in
a highly absorbent part of your body! Try these low tox options:

* Replace your current pads and tampons with organic, pure-cotton ones.
* Buy washable reusable pads and bamboo undies with the technology to
  hold onto your flow.
* Try medical-grade silicone menstrual cups. It might take a while to get
  used to them, but you buy them once for the same price as 3 months'
  worth of tampons. And you only need to change them every 12 hours.

TALK TO YOUR HEALTHCARE PROFESSIONAL

The information in this book is based on research and
expert experience I've picked up on my travels so far.
For your specific case, I *always* recommend that you see
a health practitioner to discuss your situation and goals.
Nothing compares to focused one-on-one time with
a great practitioner.

HAIR CARE

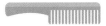

You know the major nasties we're looking to avoid now,
so there's no need to go there again.

SHAMPOO AND CONDITIONER

• • • • • •

Many natural shampoos and conditioners cost ridiculous amounts of money
if you ask me. We all have different scalps, hair types and lengths, and
desired outcomes, so I won't lie: this category will involve a bit of trial and
error over time.

NO SHAMPOO

'No poo' is the cheapest option of all. It works on the principle that after
a month or so our natural oils settle down and our hair starts to look
healthy and happy – we did, after all, manage without shampoo until the
20th century. It's not for everyone, but many who've tried it haven't looked
back. The hardest part is getting through that initial settling-down period.

Fun fact: Instructions for shampooing hair published in 1908 by
The New York Times suggested using Castile soap every two weeks
after a thorough brushing and singeing of split ends.

Alternatively, using apple cider vinegar to wash your hair (see page 76) is a way to gently remove greasiness. Simply massage in and rinse. (Seriously!)

SIMPLE HOMEMADE SHAMPOO

MAKES about 250 ml (9 fl oz/1 cup)

If you want to have a go at a DIY shampoo to see if it suits you, try this.

½ teaspoon olive oil (moisturising for dry hair) or castor oil (for oily hair)

15 drops essential oils of your choice (see note)

125 ml (4 fl oz/½ cup) distilled water (see note)

½ teaspoon xanthan gum (optional)

125 ml (4 fl oz/½ cup) Castile soap

Mix the olive or castor oil, essential oils and water in a blender for two or three pulses. With the blender running, add the xanthan gum (if using) through the top until the mixture thickens. This will take no more than 5 seconds, so watch it. Add the Castile soap and pulse just once or twice, so as not to encourage it bubbling up. Pop in an old bottle (such as a Castile soap squeezy bottle) and use when you need it, as normal.

Notes: Rosemary essential oil is a brilliant hair tonic oil as well as being invigorating at the start of the day. Using distilled water prevents mould growing in your shampoo. The xanthan gum makes a thicker, emulsified shampoo.

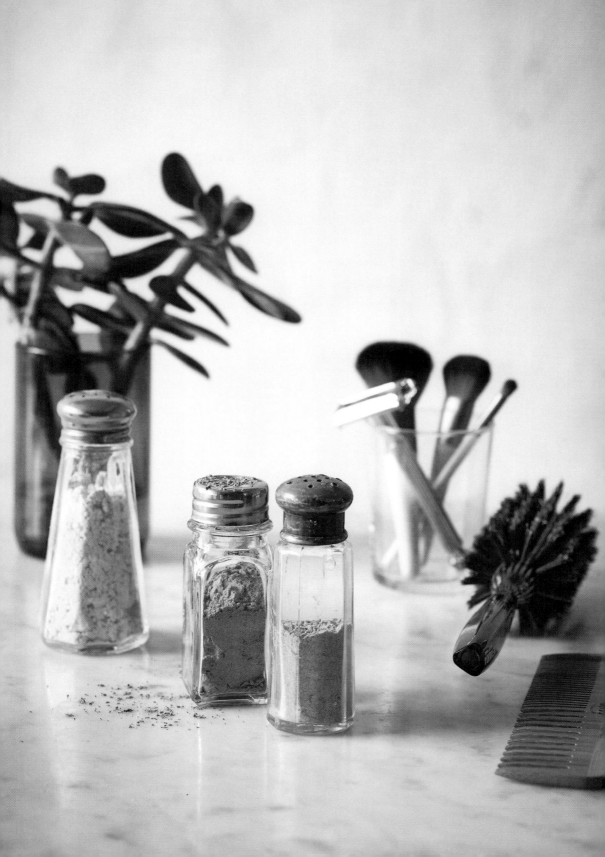

DRY SHAMPOO

MAKES 50 g (1¾ oz)

Making dry shampoo is super complicated ;-). All you need is some clean salt and pepper shaker bottles, and you're away!

BLONDE

45 g (1½ oz/⅓ cup) tapioca or arrowroot flour (see note)

1 teaspoon ground ginger

REDHEAD

45 g (1½ oz/⅓ cup) tapioca or arrowroot flour

1–2 teaspoons ground cinnamon

BRUNETTE

45 g (1½ oz/⅓ cup) tapioca or arrowroot flour

1–3 teaspoons cacao powder

Mix in a small bowl and transfer to a shaker bottle.

To use: Keep your hair dry and then after your shower – so that it won't mess up your clothes – bend forward, turning your head upside down, and dust all around the roots, then give your head a good scratch to disperse it fully. Repeat if needed.

Note: Arrowroot flour can contain E220, a preservative that can cause breathing difficulties, hives and other allergic reactions, so check the label.

TREATMENT AND STYLING PRODUCTS

• • • • • •

There's a lot we can do to treat and style our hair by way of DIY preparations straight from nature's garden. DIY isn't for everyone, and as I've said I'm definitely a mix of both DIY and bought products, so do visit lowtoxlife.com/book-resources if you fancy some help with your shopping.

HAIRSPRAY

MAKES about 125 ml (4 fl oz/½ cup)

It might seem odd to put sugar in your hair, but it works really well! If you don't need a strong hold, drop the sugar quantity back to 1 teaspoon.

125 ml (4 fl oz/½ cup) just-boiled distilled water (see note)

2 teaspoons white or rapadura sugar

1 teaspoon sea salt (optional)

1 teaspoon vanilla extract (optional)

5 drops essential oils of your choice (optional)

Mix all the ingredients together and pour into a little amber spray bottle. Spray on hair and style as usual.

Notes: Using distilled water prevents mould growing in your hairspray. The salt adds extra texture to hair.

LOW TOX HAIRBRUSHES AND TOOLS

Heat and plastic aren't a great combination when it comes to drying your hair, so go for brushes and combs made from natural materials. Ceramics and metals are best for your hair. With tools such as dryers and straightening wands, avoid plastics that come into direct contact with the heat, and avoid PFOA/PTFE (Teflon)-coated (nonstick) products.

HAIR COLOUR

· · · · · ·

This is definitely a category where unless you're using natural enhancements such as henna or cassia, for full-coverage hair colour we can only aim for 'low tox'. I really, really like my hair coloured, so for me it's a matter of making an informed choice of the least toxic option and being happy with all the other things I do in my day-to-day life as a low toxer. Some purists will disagree. That's totally fine. I take my low tox shampoo and finishing oil to the hairdresser to follow the colour, and she uses a specific colouring brand that's lower tox than mainstream salon colours. This is my way of finding peace with the situation. You're also bound to have your 'thing' where you think, 'Nope, I'm not letting that go,' so relax – our bodies can handle the odd assault. It's the daily barrage we're getting rid of here.

Foils and balayage are both great ways to avoid scalp contact during the 'taking' phase of the colour development, and can offer a good happy medium if you want to keep colouring your hair too.

DIY HOME HAIR TREATMENTS

· · · · · ·

1. **Volumising, thickening and shine:** Eggs make the perfect homemade treatment to repair and nourish hair. To use, apply 1–2 whisked eggs to clean, damp hair. Leave on for 20 minutes, then rinse with cool to mildly warm water (you don't want the egg to 'cook' – that wouldn't be too pretty!). Shampoo and condition hair as usual.

2. **Moisturising:** Coconut oil is a great treatment for super-dry hair or dry scalp and lots of frizz. Massage a couple of tablespoons through your hair and into your scalp, leave it in for 1 hour, then wash it out by shampooing twice. A double wash is definitely needed here, followed by

what you'd normally do. For dandruff, add 1 tablespoon raw honey. Add 5 drops rosemary essential oil as a tonic if you fancy.

3 **Revitalising and regenerating:** Alma powder is a brilliant strengthener and revitaliser for the hair. Simply dissolve 2 teaspoons in 1 tablespoon water. Add the juice of 1 lemon and apply to wet, clean hair. Leave in for 30 minutes. Rinse with warm water. Great for adding shine.

4 **Removing build-up:** Mix 60 ml (2 fl oz/¼ cup) apple cider vinegar with 500 ml (17 fl oz/2 cups) warm filtered water. Use in place of shampoo, scrub scalp, and finish with a cold rinse to close up cuticles.

5 **Feeding and strengthening:** Try making the recipe below. Think of it as your natural keratin treatment too if your hair is 'crazy'.

PROTEIN STRENGTHENER FOR BRITTLE HAIR

MAKES 1 treatment for long hair, 2–3 treatments for short hair

This homemade gelatine hair mask is so good. Give it a whirl if your hair needs serious resurrecting!

1 tablespoon powdered gelatine

¼ teaspoon xanthan gum (optional; see note)

125 ml (4 fl oz/½ cup) filtered water

1 teaspoon apple cider vinegar

2 teaspoons coconut milk (optional; see note)

Mix the gelatine and xanthan gum (if using) with the water in a small saucepan over medium–low heat, stirring until dissolved. Add the vinegar and coconut milk (if using). Apply to your hair between shampooing and conditioning, leaving for 2–10 minutes before rinsing thoroughly.

Note: Add the coconut milk for extra moisturising and the xanthan gum for a thicker mixture that's a bit easier to apply.

KIDS' HAIR AND THE DREADED LICE

· · · · · ·

It will perhaps come as no surprise that there's some nasty business in conventional lice treatments, but it's the simplest of things to whip up your own treatment that will kill the little bastards!

LICE TREATMENT

MAKES 1 treatment

1½ tablespoons natural shampoo

3 teaspoons coconut oil

1 teaspoon tea-tree oil

2 tablespoons conditioner

Mix the shampoo, coconut oil and tea-tree oil together in a bowl (if your coconut oil is hard, melt it first). Apply gently throughout the hair, then cover with a shower cap or towel and leave for 30 minutes.

Rinse out with warm water and then massage the 2 tablespoons of conditioner into the hair and scalp. With the conditioner in the hair, use a fine lice comb to remove the dead lice and their eggs. Rinse the hair thoroughly.

Repeat this treatment 1 week later, to ensure any eggs that didn't go in the first treatment don't get ideas about hatching and setting up camp!

NAIL CARE

With nails there are a few new things to become aware of. We're leaving behind mani-pedis at the nail place – they're most often toxic clouds of badness, and to be avoided.

After a week or two away from those places, you'll really notice how toxic the air in them is. Read on for what to avoid and what you can use instead.

THE FIVE MAIN NAIL POLISH NASTIES

● ● ● ● ● ●

1 **Dibutyl phthalate (DBP):** Pesky little phthalates! A possible trigger for asthma attacks, this phthalate has also been associated with developmental and reproductive effects, and cancer in lab animal testing. This has been called, 'a potent hormone disruptor that affects the male reproductive system most dramatically'. No, thanks!

2 **Toluene:** We met this earlier. It's a solvent, also found in some petrols, that can cause dizziness and short-term intoxication. Like DBP, it's a volatile chemical that can be inhaled and absorbed through the skin and nails.

3 **Formaldehyde:** Considered a human carcinogen by US health agencies and used to preserve animal tissue in bottles, it's an irritating chemical that causes allergic reactions. Can also be listed as 'formalin'.

4 **Formaldehyde resin:** This synthetic resin product is made with formaldehyde as a base ingredient.

5 **Camphor:** Although it can be plant-derived, this toxic compound is often synthesised from oil of turpentine, and can bring about dizziness, lethargy, asthma and rashes.

Nail polishes labelled '3-free' don't have the first three of these ingredients, while '5-free' nail polishes are missing all of them. A nail polish labelled '7-free' is free from all of the above, plus parabens, xylene, animal products and animal testing. The 7-free nail polishes do still contain some ethyl acetate (see below).

NAIL POLISH ALTERNATIVES

A super low tox nail polish option is a water-based style, although these aren't as high-performance or chip-proof, so I find you're better off making your natural nails shine through by buffing and filing. It might just be that you fall in love with well-manicured nude nails. I certainly have, and now paint only my toenails and only in the summer time, sometimes.

If having manicured nails is a top priority for you and something you're not prepared to cave on, then a 5- or 7-free brand is still a high-performance low tox compromise, and brands readily state their 'freeness' on packaging.

Acrylic nails? You have the use of methyl methacrylate (MMA), which can cause serious damage to the lungs as well as permanent damage to your natural nails. Nurses aren't allowed to wear acrylics in most countries because acrylic nail-wearers are prone to nail-bed infections from bacteria that have caused death in infants in hospitals. Lastly, due to the highly flammable nature of the adhesives, acrylic nail wearers are advised to stay away from curling and straightening irons and wands. Yikes! Might that just be the thing that tips it for you?

Shellac? Between the UVA rays and the acetone, shellac isn't recommended either. Time to move on.

NAIL POLISH REMOVER

· · · · · ·

Pure lemongrass essential oil is a good low tox nail polish remover. Place 1–2 drops on each nail, leave for 1 minute, then rub off with a little bit of elbow grease.

When buying a nail polish remover, go for the best of a bad bunch and avoid the acetone. This clear, harsh-smelling and highly flammable liquid is a solvent, capable of disintegrating even plastic. This explains why it works so quickly at breaking apart and removing your nail polish, right? The key active ingredient in non-acetone removers is usually ethyl acetate. Made from ethanol and acetic acid, ethyl acetate is a colourless and flammable solvent. It's not ideal, but if it's once in a while, if your nails are going to be 'your thing', it's a step up from acetone.

DELICIOUS NAIL TREATMENT FOR STRENGTHENING AND GROWTH

MAKES 1 treatment

All I'm going to say here is you *must* try this.

80 ml (2½ fl oz/⅓ cup) olive oil

1 tablespoon lemon juice

1 tablespoon honey

1 teaspoon sea salt

3 drops myrrh essential oil or
   tea-tree oil (see note)

Mix all the ingredients together. Soak your nails for 10 minutes. Wash with soap and dry.

Note: Tea-tree oil will give the treatment a little antibacterial and antiviral boost if you feel you need it.

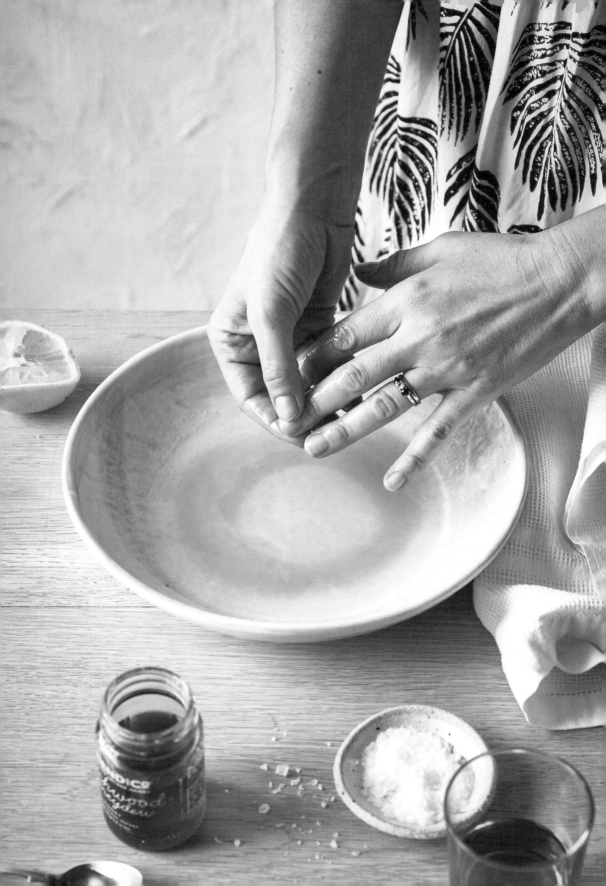

TOOTH CARE

Bless them, I love that one of the toothpaste big brands says, 'None of our toothpastes contain sugar.' As soon as a company proclaims that a product is 'something-free', ask yourself this simple question: 'So what *is* in it then?' It will save you from a lot of weirdness.

How about we look at the ingredients in the bestselling toothpastes:

* **Sodium lauryl sulfate:** It can be derived from petroleum or palm oil, can penetrate the skin and is absolutely not fine to be scrubbing into our gums, given it's a known irritant.
* **Glycerin:** The issue with glycerin is that it most often comes from unsustainable palm sources. Check your product.
* **Sodium saccharin:** This petroleum-derived chemical, added to make the toothpaste taste sweet, is suspected of reproductive and developmental toxicity, and can cause rash and hives.
* **Flavour:** Whatever that means ... This can be artificial, can be real, can be toxic, can be not. Problem is, *what* is it? It's an umbrella term for so many things, and we don't like mystery.
* **Triclosan:** We're old hands at this 'antibacterial, chloroform off-gassing number' now, aren't we?
* **Microbeads.** Yep, again! Tens of thousands of BPA-containing plastic fragments, headed to a waterway near you every time we brush. Isn't that just crazy? Would you pick up a bunch of tiny blue beads, scrub them into your teeth and go, 'Ahhh, just what I needed for tartar control'? Didn't think so. Let the weirdness end today!

THE REAL SECRET TO PREVENTING TOOTH DECAY

Weston A. Price, a dentist in the 1930s, devoted a decade of his life to studying traditional cultures that were eating traditional unprocessed foods. His book, *Nutrition and Physical Degeneration*, is fascinating. He concluded that cultures that hadn't been introduced to refined grains and sugar, and ate a traditional diet of whatever 'their people' ate (everything from blubber to raw cream, sourdough, vegetarian, cultured foods, liver and more) showed little tooth decay, if any.

After 40 years of practice, my wonderful dentist, Dr Ron Ehrlich, insists that the most powerful preventative for tooth decay is diet. 'A diet of real, nutrient-dense and colourful natural food, with minimal to no refined and processed foods, gets you a long way to feeling awesome and having strong teeth. This will help prevent tooth decay in the most powerful way possible.'

Focusing on mineral-rich food and fat-soluble vitamins A, D, E and K – which ensure minerals get to your teeth – will do much more for you than fluoride, although this can be useful sometimes, applied topically when there is decay.

NATURAL TOOTH-CARE OPTIONS

· · · · · ·

If you want to explore the natural side of things when it comes to your teeth, try these alternatives:

✳ **Toothpaste:** Find a good natural one that doesn't have those key nasties in it, and you'll be getting the clean without the yikes! You could mix up a simple DIY toothpaste with 2 tablespoons coconut oil, 25 g (1 oz) calcium carbonate, 10 drops peppermint oil and 1 drop clove oil. Store in a clean small pot.

✳ **Mouthwash:** There are some awesome natural mouthwashes out there without artificial colours, flavours, sweeteners or alcohol. To make your own, dilute 3 drops peppermint oil, 1 drop cinnamon oil and 1 drop clove oil in ½ teaspoon olive oil, and mix with 125 ml (4 fl oz/½ cup) distilled water. Shake well before use.

✳ **Whitening:** Activated charcoal is an excellent gradual whitener, as is a hydrogen peroxide gel, but *only* under the guidance of your dentist.

✳ **Floss:** Seek out a silk floss, because most flosses are coated in – wait for it – PTFEs (Teflon), and the floss itself is a synthetic of some kind, often nylon. Given that Americans use around 4.3 million kilometres of floss annually, it stands to reason we'd want to substitute something that doesn't release PTFEs, which never break down, into the environment.

✳ **Tongue cleaner:** The Ayurvedic tradition is to scrape the tongue upon waking to remove toxins and bad bugs that may have accumulated in the mouth overnight. It's strangely addictive is all I can say. I use a stainless-steel scraper.

✳ **Toothbrush:** A bamboo brush is the most environmentally friendly choice. It's a great option – especially for little kiddies or sensitive teeth, as the bristles are quite soft.

PERSONAL FRAGRANCE

Most 'prestige' perfume is full of fake stuff, unfortunately.
A couple of more traditional houses use essential oils for their
classic perfumes, but it's extremely rare, and most contain
synthetics, with phthalates most often hiding in there to help
the perfume last. If you're unsure, ask the company.

I've worn natural fragrance for about eight years now, and I honestly
can't believe how strongly the fake ones smell, and nor can I get my head
around how exactly I was able to wear them, let alone proudly manage the
fragrance counter at the local duty-free one summer during university! At
the time and into my next few years in the beauty industry, I had migraines
twice a week, but I never made the connection until I left cosmetics and
the migraines disappeared. I still remember the lovely friend who ran the
Clarins counter lending me her beauty room to sleep the migraine off a
bit with heavy painkillers while the manager was off for lunch. It's amazing
how quickly you realise synthetic fragrances smell really wrong once you've
removed them from your day-to-day life.

   If we could just go back and speak to our past selves, right? 'Join the dots,
girl, *join the dots*!

*It's amazing how quickly you realise synthetic
fragrances smell really wrong.*

NATURAL FRAGRANCE IDEAS

• • • • • •

Seek out natural brands and try a few over the next few months. This is
a great category for the Christmas and birthday lists.

Tip: Many brands with multiple natural fragrances offer trial vials at a tiny
cost, so you can try before you commit to sizes more than 50 ml (1¾ fl oz).

DIY FRAGRANCE WITH OILS

• • • • • •

It's amazing how many people have stopped me to ask what I was wearing
when it was just a drop of vetiver oil behind the ears. This is a simple, natural
and, per drop, generally very inexpensive (although oils from certain plants
with lower yields are, of course, more expensive). There are many essential
oil companies out there. Just do your research and ensure the oils are
pure and unadulterated, that the company tests them in house as well as
independently, and that their distilling and farming methods are transparent
and sustainable. It takes a lot of raw material to produce an essential oil, so
you want to ensure they're not abusing nature.

When it comes to making your own blends, you can work on the principle
of including a head note, heart note and base note, just as the great
perfumers of the past did. In a 10 ml (⅓ fl oz) roll-on bottle, do 9 ml carrier
oil such as almond oil and then 5 drops of your head note, 10 drops of
your heart note and 15 of your base note. Play with your favourite singles,
following the pyramid opposite as a guideline. My current favourite is
2 drops each of ginger and rosemary as my head note, 6 drops neroli and
2 of jasmine as my heart note, and 10 drops spruce and 5 drops vetiver as
my base note. Into the roll-on and off we go! Quite sexy, if I do say so myself.

PERFUME PYRAMID

● ● ● ● ● ●

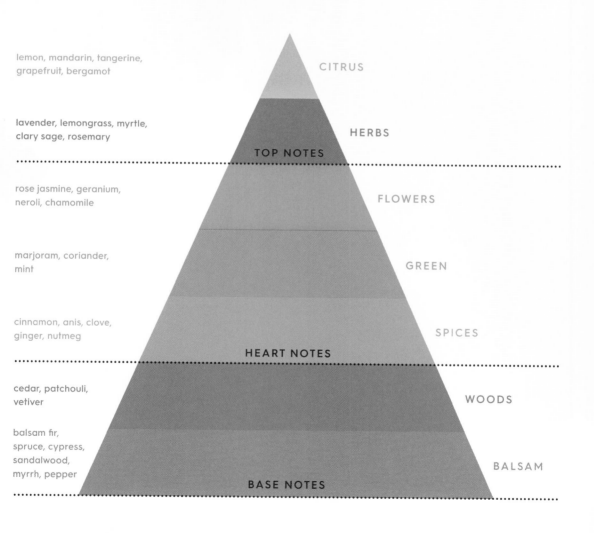

lemon, mandarin, tangerine,
grapefruit, bergamot

CITRUS

lavender, lemongrass, myrtle,
clary sage, rosemary

HERBS

TOP NOTES

rose jasmine, geranium,
neroli, chamomile

FLOWERS

marjoram, coriander,
mint

GREEN

cinnamon, anis, clove,
ginger, nutmeg

SPICES

HEART NOTES

cedar, patchouli,
vetiver

WOODS

balsam fir,
spruce, cypress,
sandalwood,
myrrh, pepper

BALSAM

BASE NOTES

BODY

SIMPLE DETOX SOLUTIONS

You might start thinking: 'Well, hold on. How do we get the stuff *out* of our bodies that's already in there?'

What you've been doing bit by bit, since you started reading this book and making changes, is detoxing without even doing a thing other than ceasing to use certain substances in your day-to-day life. Your body is clever. To really start to rid it of some of the 'stickier' chemicals that reside inside us – especially in our fat tissues and organs – as a result of having used all these products over the years, you can choose to embark upon what I call a Conscious Detox Process. It's not what you might think. You won't be starving yourself or having to do a juice fast for 5 days.

Only when you're mentally positive and relaxed will you truly start to feel the benefits of detoxification of any kind.

The key is to be gentle with yourself, and support the detoxification your body already does with lots of low tox mind time (see Chapter 5) as well. Only when you're mentally positive and relaxed will you truly start to feel the benefits of detoxification of any kind. It makes sense, really. If you're stressed, your body draws energy away from your digestive detox pathways and immune system to use all your energy on 'saving your life'. So calm down, take those nature walks, and get ready to detox the right way, every day, little bit by little bit, as our bodies are designed to.

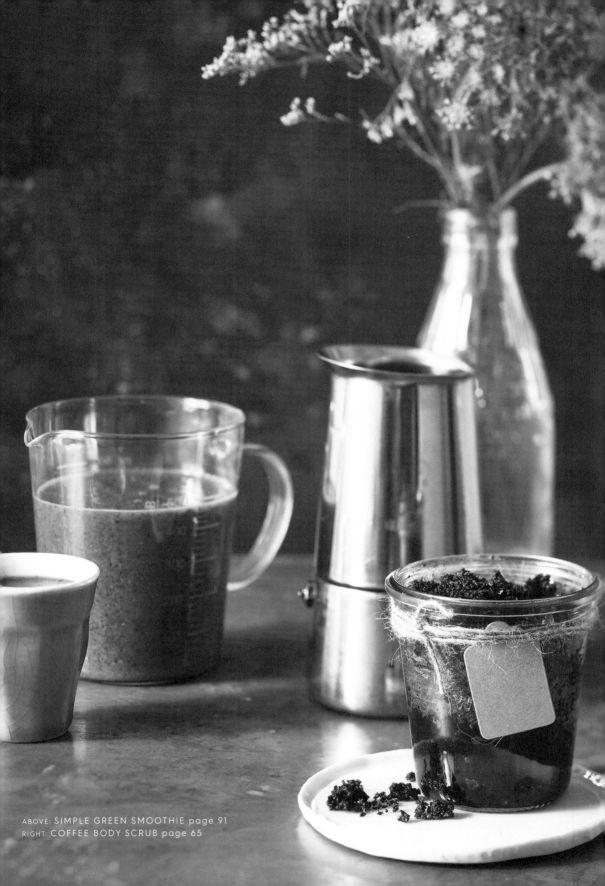

ABOVE: SIMPLE GREEN SMOOTHIE page 91
RIGHT: COFFEE BODY SCRUB page 65

SIMPLE DETOX IDEAS

• • • • • •

Here are some simple ideas to road-test. Make an appointment with a doctor or naturopath to decide together what your best detox support could be.

* **Stop applying and ingesting nasties in the first place:** You're already blitzing detox by not using all the stuff you used to.

* **Consider taking a break from harder-to-digest foods:** Some foods are known to be more difficult to digest, so try avoiding them for a short period of time, such as a month. This could include one or all of gluten, dairy, nuts, unfermented soy and eggs. It's a great break for the system.

* **Eat organic where possible:** Some pesticide constituents are endocrine-disruptive (see Chapter 4), so minimising pesticide residues is helpful.

* **Eat more vegetables:** It's so simple, yet brings such a massive increase in micronutrients, promoting health at the cellular level, enabling your body to do its job better.

* **Use a good body scrub:** This has a similar effect to my Coffee Body Scrub (page 65) – make your own in minutes!

A NOTE FOR PREGNANT WOMEN

Do not undertake any extreme detoxification when pregnant or breastfeeding. From the list above, regular dry brushing, massage, a carrot salad and my suggested very gentle chelating herb smoothie (on the opposite page) are plenty to be doing while pregnant or breastfeeding. And always discuss these with your health practitioner first.

* **Take baths with Epsom salts, MSM, clay and/or magnesium flakes:** Just 15–20 minutes will ensure some of these powerful detoxifiers seep into your skin *or* draw toxins *out* of your skin. Spray a little magnesium oil under your feet as you get out. Bliss!

* **Consider an enema or a round of colonics.**

* **Eat foods that chelate:** In other words, they bind to heavy metals and other toxins, and draw them out of the body. There's a lot of research on coriander (cilantro) to suggest it can assist with heavy metal detoxification. Try making a simple green smoothie with 250 ml (9 fl oz/ 1 cup) water, 125 ml (4 fl oz/½ cup) coconut water or chilled herbal tea, ½ bunch coriander, ½ cucumber and the juice of 1 lime, whizzed in a good blender for 1 minute. This is two serves for two days.

* **Use a dry body brush before your shower:** Brushing is traditionally thought to stimulate the lymphatic system.

* **Eat a simple raw carrot salad in the morning:** Season 80 g (2¾ oz/ ½ cup) raw grated carrot with apple cider vinegar, lemon and olive oil. It's extremely cleansing and a great morning detox kickstart. Thanks to friend and holistic practitioner Shalani McCray for that one.

* **Do yoga:** Poses with twists and releases can 'flush out' your organs.

* **Get a deep tissue massage:** Stimulate the shift of toxins from your tissues. Be sure to drink a couple of glasses of water or herbal tea afterwards, to support the process.

* **Experiment with 'binders':** Talk to your health practitioner about trying diatomaceous earth, charcoal, bentonite clay and/or zeolites.

* **Try oil pulling:** This ancient Ayurvedic dental technique involves swishing 1 tablespoon oil (preferably coconut oil or cold-pressed sesame oil) around your mouth on an empty stomach for about 20 minutes. This action is said to draw out toxins in the body, primarily to improve oral health, but also overall health. To be honest, it makes me nauseous, but my very experienced dentist highly recommends it. It's up to you!

* **Do movement that makes you sweat, at least five times a week.**

CHAPTER THREE

· · · · · · ·

LOW TOX
HOME

BREATHING EASY
AT HOME

It's our right to feel safest in our own house, and this pillar of the Low Tox Life is about bringing a beautiful sense of what's good and true into our homes, and letting go of what's not.

If you go to the supermarket for a multipurpose spray or washing liquid, or buy a mattress or computer cable, it's actually very hard to find out the ingredients or components. Why? They're not required to list them by law unless there's a known hazard in the mix (think drain cleaner listing sodium hydroxide or bleach listing its percentage). The problem with that is that testing isn't demanded of all chemicals that are registered for use, and that 'hazard' most often means immediate impacts such as burning, lung irritation or skin damage. We know from Chapter 2 that chemicals have many effects that aren't front-page news – some very quiet, some cumulative over time at the lowest of levels, and some even having intergenerational effects through genetic modulation. You're not going to see any time soon on your washing powder 'Warning: This fragrance contains phthalates. Potential risk to sexual development of male infants and interference with the endocrine system' or on your tinned beans lined with BPA 'Warning: Your grandchild may have altered genetics due to your BPA exposure'.

Regulatory bodies around the world largely leave the onus on the chemical company to ensure the safety of their products and to register their chemicals with the regulator. Given the speed with which new chemicals

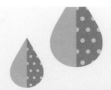

come to market, the regulators don't have the people power to validate research or conduct extensive studies of their own, and it's due to these inadequate regulatory set-ups that we have the basic situation today of a chemical essentially being innocent until proven guilty. Regulatory bodies are also, unfortunately, often beholden in part to the chemical industry they regulate. The degree to which this occurs varies from country to country, but it's a contributing factor to the lack of safety in our stuff. While money can influence Bills, Acts and policy through artful lobbying, it will be impossible to achieve subjective regulation of chemicals. The American 2009 Endocrine Disruption Prevention Bill aimed to move the responsibility for research away from the Environmental Protection Agency to the National Institute of Environmental Health Sciences, which is not influenced by industry. The Bill failed to be passed. We stay vigilant.

It's all about your priorities, and there's no perfect way to do low tox other than your way.

Given we have very little way of finding out what's in many mainstream household items and very little guarantee that extensive safety testing has been done on short- and long-term uses, and low- and high-level exposure, on all systems of the body, the best we can do is seek out the companies that are leading the charge in transparency and green chemistry. Another alternative, if it's your thing, is to get your DIY on. As I've said before, I'm very much a mix of both, making a few of my own things and supporting sustainable brands. It's all about your priorities, and there's no perfect way to do low tox other than your way.

So in this section we're going to look at the home. We'll discover some simple and effective home-cleaning and laundry recipes. We'll learn ways to minimise our exposure to electromagnetic fields (without having to give up our technology), volatile organic compounds (VOCs) and plastics. We'll find out how to reduce phthalate exposure and lung irritants through our home-fragrance choices. And how to develop more sustainable attitudes with textiles, ensure better water quality and – my personal favourite, and something I'm still working hard on – own less stuff.

MENTAL LOW-TOX HEALTH CHECK

✓ Remember that this isn't a race.

✓ Start with whatever strikes you as the most urgent for you, not someone else. Having a strong sense of why is critical to helping you feel these changes are possible.

✓ Celebrate every small change rather than lamenting everything you didn't know before.

✓ Involve your family in the learning process with the documentaries and resources suggested at lowtoxlife.com/book-resources.

✓ Remind yourself that stressing about what hasn't changed yet or what you see around you won't serve you. Let it go. Focus on the change you're making. Let the ripples from that change do their work in time.

CLEANING AND LAUNDRY PRODUCTS

The issue with nasty cleaning products is that not only do they pollute us and our waterways, but they can severely compromise our indoor air quality. Be prepared to have fresher air than ever in your home haven from this moment onwards.

CHEMICALS TO AVOID

• • • • • •

Here we go on the major nasties found in common cleaning products. If they don't list them on the bottle, that tends to be all the confirmation I need to avoid it. The standard reason is that their ingredients are a 'proprietary blend', but many great companies with nothing to hide list theirs, and the gift of the chemist is in the ratios and blending, which easily remains proprietary, whether there's a visible ingredients list or not.

Once you've seen one nasty on there, there's no point trying to make out what all the other chemicals are … You've already decided. Over time, you'll find the simpler natural options and brands you can trust. I've shared mine here too, and some super-easy DIY recipes if you prefer to make your own or need a budget-friendly option. Or you can find some great brand suggestions over at lowtoxlife.com/book-resources.

PHTHALATES (PARTICULARLY DIETHYL PHTHALATE)

We find these in air fresheners, synthetically fragranced cleaning products, many scented candles, household furnishings, PVC flooring, and food packaging such as plastic wrap and freezer bags.

✗ Health risk: They are endocrine disruptive to varying degrees. You'll only see 'fragrance' on a label, so think again when you see scent claims such as 'spring fresh' or 'rainforest'. I don't know about you, but I find these products smell very different from the real thing they claim to be mimicking.

TRICLOSAN

Petroleum-derived, originally classed as a pesticide in 1969, triclosan is the bad boy behind the 'antibacterial' craze, and is often used in cleaning products, hand soap, deodorant, antibacterial face washes and toothpastes.

✗ Health risks: Triclosan can disrupt the immune system and accumulate in the environment. Studies have called for urgent further research into its toxic effects on certain algae and fish. How is it still allowed to be used so widely? Lack of regulation is how, but thankfully we're finally gaining some traction with this chemical. Canada declared it toxic to the environment in 2012, and the United States ordered it to be removed from hand sanitisers and liquid soaps in 2017.

2-BUTOXYETHANOL

This chemical gives window, kitchen and multipurpose cleaners their characteristic sweet smell. It belongs in the category of glycol ethers, a set of powerful solvents that don't mess around. Manufacturers are not required to list 2-butoxyethanol on a product's label.

✗ Health risks: In addition to causing lung irritation when inhaled, at high levels, glycol ethers can contribute to narcosis (sleepiness), pulmonary oedema (fluid in the lungs), and severe liver and kidney damage. Dr Rebecca Sutton, a senior scientist for the Environmental Working Group (EWG), warns, 'Although the EPA sets a standard on 2-butoxyethanol for workplace safety, you can actually end up getting 2-butoxyethanol in the air at levels that are higher than workplace safety standards.'

AMMONIA

Because ammonia evaporates and doesn't leave streaks, it's another common ingredient in commercial window cleaners.

✗ Health risks: That sparkle has a price. 'Ammonia is a powerful irritant,' says Donna Kasuska, a chemical engineer and president of ChemConscious, Inc., a risk-management consulting company. 'It's going to affect you right away. The people who will be really affected are those who have asthma, and elderly people with lung issues and breathing problems. It's almost always inhaled. People who get a lot of ammonia exposure, like housekeepers, will often develop chronic bronchitis and asthma.' Ammonia can also create poisonous chloramine gas if it's mixed with bleach.

✓ Healthier choice: White vinegar or vodka. Vodka will 'produce a reflective shine on any metal or mirrored surface.' So pour a vodka soda and do some window cleaning. Doesn't sound all that bad now, does it?

CHLORINE

We find it mainly in scouring powders, toilet cleaners, whiteners for laundry soaking and cleaning, mould-removal products, tap water and pool water. You're getting exposed through fumes and possibly through the skin when you clean with it, but because it's also in town water to get rid of bacteria, you're also getting exposed when you take a shower or bath or drink tap water or, of course, when you swim in a chlorinated pool.

✗ Health risks: These can be acute (sudden) or chronic (long term). Chlorine can affect the eyes, skin and respiratory system.

SODIUM HYDROXIDE

Found in some oven cleaners and drain openers.

✗ Health risks: Also called lye, sodium hydroxide is extremely corrosive. If it touches your skin or gets in your eyes, it can cause severe burns, and inhaling the stuff can cause a sore throat that lasts for days. If you dread using oven cleaner, your instinct was right and you've found the reason why. This stuff is horrible.

SODIUM LAURETH SULFATE

A surfactant, detergent, and emulsifier used in thousands of cosmetic products, as well as in industrial cleaners. It's present in most mainstream shampoos, scalp treatments, hair colour and bleaching agents, toothpastes, body washes and cleansers, make-up foundations, liquid hand soaps, laundry detergents and bath gels. It can be manufactured from coconuts, but it's more damaging to the environment when it's manufactured from unsustainable palm oil or petroleum.

✗ Health risk: A real problem with sodium laureth sulfate is that the manufacturing process (ethoxylation) results in it being contaminated with 1,4-dioxane, a carcinogenic by-product.

Note: Sodium *lauryl* sulfate, while not to be used on skin or in personal care due to its potential as a skin irritant, is a better option for cleaning if it's made from coconut oil or sustainable palm oil. It's not carcinogenic and doesn't contain any 1,4-dioxane as a by-product. It's handy, as it does dissolve tough stains and grime from the grout in bathrooms very well.

PETROLEUM DISTILLATES (AKA NAPTHAS)

Found in most mainstream laundry detergents and softeners.

✗ Health risks: Napthas, depending on regularity and degree of exposure, can irritate the respiratory system and possibly the kidneys. They can also be contaminated with benzene, a known carcinogen.

PHOSPHATES

You know how you see a 'P' or an 'NP' on laundry powder or detergent packaging? Well, the P stands for phosphates. They stimulate the growth of certain marine plants when they're released into the environment, and contribute to unbalanced ecosystems. Every dollar we spend, we *do* have a chance to contribute to a better world.

OPTICAL BRIGHTENERS

Found in laundry detergents. Safety data sheets for multiple brighteners clearly show their toxicity to aquatic life, and they can cause bacterial mutations and allergic reactions.

QUATERNARY AMMONIUM COMPOUNDS (QUATS)

Found in fabric softeners and fabric-softening sheets, as well as many shampoos, conditioners and face and body products.

✗ Health risks: These operate similarly to triclosan and, to boot, can cause asthma and dermatitis.

OTHER SUBSTANCES IN FABRIC SOFTENERS

Fabric softeners also commonly contain benzyl acetate (possibly linked to pancreatic cancer), benzyl alcohol (can irritate the respiratory system depending on the source of its raw materials) and chloroform (a neurotoxin and carcinogen). To top it off, many of them are petroleum-based, which takes a toll on a non-renewable resource and is non-biodegradable.

PALM OIL

This deforestation disaster ingredient kills innocent orangutan populations throughout South-East Asia when their rainforest habitat is destroyed to make way for palm plantations. It's essential to ensure your laundry products – if they do contain palm oil – are from a certified sustainable farm. We must start to pressure our brands for traceable sustainability from their suppliers too. A handful around the world are doing the right thing. Ecostore and Dr Bronner's, for example, can both attest to that, and you can request sustainability certification from other brands too. If you feel passionate about palm oil issues, Palmoil Investigations (POI) is a great resource, and has an app that scans barcodes to tell you which products contain palm oil.

DIY OPTIONS YOU CAN USE INSTEAD

· · · · · · ·

Let's start this with ditching just one thing in your home, like fabric softener. It excites me to goosebump levels that our indoor air pollution will plummet from this moment forward in homes where conventional mainstream fabric softener has been used in the past but will be no longer. Get excited, people!

Imagine thousands of other people around the world reading this and picture all the fabric softener being retired. The thousands of kilos of toxic nasties out of circulation. And thousands of people breathing easier, being less subjected to endocrine disruption by potent synthetic fragrances. How exciting is that!

You can DIY using the recipes here or buy from the handful of companies around the world that are doing the right thing.

FIRST YOUR TOOLS

✓ Rubber, powder-free gloves.

✓ Cloths and sponges made from natural bamboo or coconut fibres, to avoid microplastic particles from microfibres going down the sink or washing-machine drain, or out into the air from your clothes dryer if you use one.

✓ Bamboo or wooden-handled cleaning brushes and scrubbers. Beautiful-quality ones are available around the world, and trading up on quality means buying less often, too, so you end up cost-neutral.

✓ Tree-free or recycled papers for kitchen paper towel, if you use it, or try reusable natural-fibre cloths and tea towels as your go-to instead.

✓ For DIY: the 'Buy nothing new' option is simply to reuse your current spray bottles and tubs, and fill them with your own recipes. If you want new, non-branded DIY supplies, invest in some amber glass spray bottles (two is plenty) and save some jars for cream cleaners and washing powders.

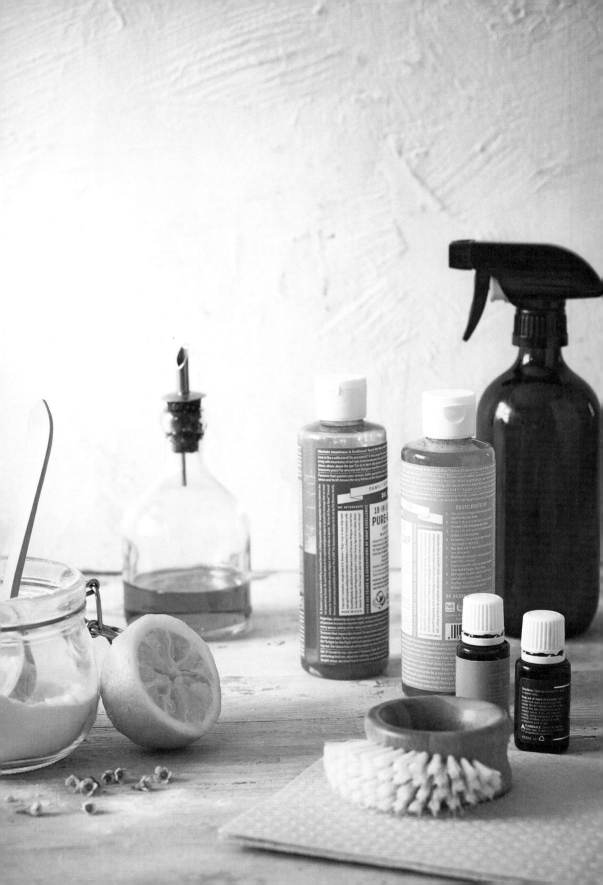

THEN YOUR INGREDIENTS

You'll be using:

- ✓ white vinegar from distilled, fermented spirit. If it doesn't specify that it's been made from distilled spirit, then it could contain petroleum.
- ✓ Castile soap
- ✓ sea salt
- ✓ bicarbonate of soda (baking soda)
- ✓ essential oils
- ✓ olive oil
- ✓ lemons
- ✓ water.

Revolutionary stuff! So simple. So inexpensive!

A NOTE ON FLOORING, SURFACES AND GREY-WATER/SEPTIC TANKS

All the DIY options here (and those from any brands mentioned) are safe for grey-water/septic tanks. If you have floors with porous surfaces, such as marble, varnished wood or cork, or marble, wood or concrete benchtops, keep the vinegar to a minimum in your DIY recipes and up the Castile soap a little instead.

MULTIPURPOSE SPRAY

Use this on kitchen surfaces, and around sinks, windowsills, mantelpieces, shower tiles. DO NOT use on wood.

250 ml (9 fl oz/1 cup) white vinegar (see note)

250 ml (9 fl oz/1 cup) water (see note)

½ teaspoon eucalyptus or tea-tree essential oil

½ teaspoon rosemary essential oil (optional)

Pop it all in a spray bottle. Shaky-shake before use. Done.

Note: If you have porous benchtops, omit the vinegar and use 1 tablespoon Castile soap, 250 ml (9 fl oz/1 cup) water and 15 drops essential oil. If you go through your bottle of multipurpose cleaner quite quickly, you can use water from the tap. Otherwise, use distilled water to prevent mould growth in the long term.

ANTIBACTERIAL SURFACE SPRAY

Make as for the Multipurpose Spray, but with 1 teaspoon extra of either eucalyptus, tea-tree or neem essential oil in the mix. Revolutionary, right?

MOULD CLEANER

Did you know that bleach doesn't kill mould? All those vapours upsetting your lungs and for what? The mould actually omits a toxic gas in retaliation against the bleach then feeds on the chlorine, and while the bleach removes it from sight, it's still alive under there and grows back.

There are two types of mould situations. There's the type that's just on the tile or surface as a result of a bit too much moisture in the room due to condensation build-up – in bathrooms or around windows in winter. These can be cleaned away with these easy DIY spray mixtures:

* **Non-porous surface:** Make up a solution of 80% white vinegar and 20% water. Clean with an old cloth. Dispose of this cloth or wash it twice, once in a bucket of 50% water and 50% white vinegar, and then in a bucket of water.

* **Porous surface:** Make up a solution of 70% any pure white alcohol and 30% water. If it's started eating away at the material already, consider replacing it.

Then there's the structural type that appears to grow from the inside of the walls or up from the flooring or down through clogged gutters. The latter needs specialised mould-remediation treatment and the root cause needs to be found and fixed. If mould is an ongoing concern for you, explore the work of Nicole Bijlsma and Dr Sandeep Gupta in the area of mould removal and health treatment respectively.

Please wear a mask when cleaning mould. Up to a quarter of the population doesn't make antibodies against mould, which means exposure wreaks havoc on their health. If you have bizarre and multiple symptoms that you can't explain or make sense of, including extreme fatigue and brain fog, explore whether you have a mould problem in your home.

STAINLESS-STEEL CLEANER

This is a tough one to make, and can get really tricky. You ready?

1 lemon, cut in half

Squeeze a little lemon juice into your morning juice or smoothie or salad dressing. Casually wipe the remaining half all over your sink, laundry sink and other stainless-steel surfaces. Then wipe down with a damp cloth. Done!

FURNITURE POLISH

FOR DARK WOOD OR LEATHER

Oh dear, another really tough one that I'm sure will make you switch straight back to those old toxic furniture polishes …

olive oil

Dab a little on a tea towel (dish towel) and really rub it in so you can't feel any oil when you wipe it with your hand. Then? Polish your couch. That's it. Seriously. Do wooden furniture, leather furniture and leather shoes with this and you'll be amazed.

Note: Test a small patch first, to ensure it suits your type of leather. DO NOT use on suede.

GLASS CLEANER

125 ml (4 fl oz/½ cup) water
60 ml (2 fl oz/¼ cup) white vinegar

4 drops cinnamon, tea-tree or peppermint essential oil (optional; see note)

Pour into a spray bottle and shake to mix. Use to clean your windows with a tea towel (dish towel) or bamboo microfibre cloth. Simple.

Note: Add the essential oil to deter critters from the outside coming in.

DISHWASHER CLEANER AND RINSE AID

You're never going to have that slippery 'sheen' to your dishes again. It was a fake. Nasty chemicals make that ultra-shiny sheen.

125 ml (4 fl oz/½ cup) white vinegar or juice of 1 lemon

Once a month, or even every fortnight, put the vinegar in a small cup in your dishwasher (NOT in the rinse aid compartment as the acid can wear the plastic down). Do a quick wash cycle. Job done.

OVEN CLEANER

This is great. So easy, and no more poisoning your lungs with those toxic cleaners and lung irritants.

65 g (2¼ oz/¼ cup) sea salt   **45 g (1½ oz/¼ cup) bicarbonate of**
60 ml (2 fl oz/¼ cup) white vinegar   **soda (baking soda)**

Turn the oven to 180°C (350°F).
Mix all the ingredients together in a jar and set aside.

Half-fill a baking dish with water, sit it in the oven and 'bake' to create steam for about 30 minutes. DO NOT add the paste to this dish.

Allow the oven to cool a little, then scrub your paste over the oven walls and door. Wipe down. Rinse with a couple of very damp tea towels (dish towels) and then a couple of dry ones. Done.

Notes: Although ¼ cup of each ingredient is good for an average-sized oven, you can simply mix equal volumes of the three ingredients to make as much of the paste as you need. Don't add an essential oil to this one. Rose-geranium baked pumpkin anyone? No, thank you, that would be a bit weird!

CREAM CLEANSER

I don't make this often, because I find that a cream cleanser isn't really needed. If it's a texture you like, however, be my guest.

95 g (3¼ oz/½ cup) bicarbonate of soda (baking soda)

1 tablespoon coarse salt

125 ml (4 fl oz/½ cup) water

10 drops essential oil of your choice (optional)

Mix the bicarbonate of soda, salt and water in a jar. If they don't form a paste, keep adding a little water, bit by bit, until they do. Add the essential oil (if using) for beautiful fragrance. Use to scrub your bath or stovetop.

FLOOR CLEANER

500 ml (17 fl oz/2 cups) water

2 tablespoons liquid Castile soap

125 ml (4 fl oz/½ cup) white vinegar (see note)

10–20 drops essential oil of your choice (see note)

1 tablespoon bicarbonate of soda (baking soda) (see note)

Combine all the ingredients in a bottle and shake a little before use.

This is enough to either do one large tiled living space, or two 'servings' for a standard kitchen floor using 1⅓ cups at a time. I use it neat, pouring it on the floor and then cleaning with a mop.

Notes: For varnished, marble and polished concrete floors, add an extra tablespoon of Castile soap and ditch the vinegar and bicarbonate of soda. The bicarbonate of soda is optional but can help lift stains from things like beetroot or turmeric. For essential oils, I like eucalyptus for disinfecting floors and a citrusy oil such as lemon myrtle or tangerine for freshness in the air, so I do a combination of 10 drops of each.

CARPET STAIN REMOVERS

Patch-test these methods on a tiny area at the edge of the carpet or rug.

1. For a bad stain (like red wine), mix a couple of tablespoons each of hydrogen peroxide (3%) and Castile soap, and rub into the stain. Leave for 10 minutes to work some magic, then rinse with water and use tea towels (dish towels) to blot dry. Repeat if needed.

2. A paste of bicarbonate of soda (baking soda) and water is also great for carpet stains. Just scrub on with a little water, leave for 30 minutes, rinse with water and blot dry. DO NOT leave on overnight or it might lighten the carpet.

BRIGHTENING SUBSTITUTE
FOR CLOTHES-WASHING OR BATHROOM SURFACES

250 ml (9 fl oz/1 cup) water

25 ml (1 fl oz) hydrogen peroxide
(3%) (see note)

20 g (¾ oz) bicarbonate of soda
(baking soda)

1 tablespoon lemon juice

5 drops lemon essential oil

Mix all the ingredients together in a 1 litre (35 fl oz/4 cup) bottle. The mixture will keep for 1 week. Don't store it longer than this, as the hydrogen peroxide can cause the mixture to expand over time.

Add ⅓ cup to your clothes washes, or work it over surfaces with a sponge for brightening up the bathroom.

Note: You can buy small bottles of 3% hydrogen peroxide in supermarkets, or buy 6% in a chemist and water it down by mixing with an equal volume of water.

JEWELLERY CLEANER

FOR SILVER, COPPER AND BRASS

This whole book is worth it for this nifty cleaning trick alone. When you see my gorgeous coffee pot in the shot with the Coffee Body Scrub (page 89), you'll know that I used this cleaner on it. It takes just a few minutes for the tarnish to disappear. You can also use it to brighten gold and white gold.

1–2 tablespoons bicarbonate of soda (baking soda)
1 teaspoon salt

Find a bowl that fits the item you want to clean, and line the bowl with aluminium foil. Place the bicarbonate of soda and salt in the bowl, then pour in enough boiling water to cover the item in question. Immerse the item in this solution and leave to clean for 5 minutes. Take out and rinse.

GROUT CLEANER

Double the quantity if you're in dire need and you have a large bathroom. Soup it up as an anti-mould grout cleaner with 1 teaspoon tea-tree oil, and always wear a mask in spaces where mould might be present.

If this doesn't clean your grout and your grout is old, it may simply need to be replaced.

65 g (2¼ oz/⅓ cup) bicarbonate of soda (baking soda)
hydrogen peroxide (3%)

Pour the bicarbonate of soda into a big glass bowl. Very slowly mix in hydrogen peroxide until the mixture forms a paste.

Scrub into the grout, leave for 30 minutes, then rinse off.

LOO CLEANER

Even when cleaning the loo we can easily avoid all the nasties with a very simple homemade formula.

95 g (3¼ oz/½ cup) bicarbonate of soda (baking soda) (see note)
10 drops good-quality eucalyptus or tea-tree oil
125 ml (4 fl oz/½ cup) white vinegar
2 tablespoons hydrogen peroxide (6%) (optional)

Sprinkle the bicarbonate of soda around the loo. Drop the oil into the toilet-bowl water. Pour the vinegar over the sprinkled bicarbonate of soda and, as it bubbles up, use your toilet brush to swirl things around and scrub, to give everything a good disinfect and clean. Leave for 20 minutes before flushing.

If your toilet bowl is a bit stained, add the hydrogen peroxide to the bowl and leave it for 30 minutes before flushing. Alternatively, go one more round with the bicarbonate of soda and vinegar.

Note: Bicarbonate of soda is magic for smelly 'situations' too. Keep an open packet behind the loo instead of those fake-smelling weirdo sprays.

LIME SCALE IN COFFEE MACHINE OR KETTLE

white vinegar or lemon juice

Your kettle is a ready-made liquid container, so the descaling process is pretty simple. Start by quarter-filling the kettle with vinegar or lemon juice and leaving for 1 hour. DO NOT boil at this stage. Leave in the vinegar or lemon juice, top up the kettle with water and boil. Pour away the boiled water before it cools, then rinse out the kettle with several changes of cold water to remove any traces of vinegar or lemon juice (not a good taste with coffee!).

To descale a coffee maker, quarter-fill the water compartment with vinegar or lemon juice, then top up with water and run the coffee-making process with this solution and no coffee. Repeat twice with plain water to rinse.

WASHING POWDER

This is a super-simple DIY recipe. Feel free to double batch it if you have a large family and do a lot of laundry. DIY might feel expensive with the initial outlay for all the ingredients, but buy in bulk and it works out to be an economical way to go in the long run.

1½ cups washing soda (sodium carbonate; see note)
1½ cups borax (sodium borate)
1 bar natural soap, finely grated (e.g. Dr Bronner's or Weleda)

Wearing gloves, carefully mix the washing soda with the borax, and then add the finely grated soap. Store in an airtight container. Use ¼ cup per load. If it's a really dirty load, add an extra tablespoon or two of borax – it's brilliant for removing fungi and bacteria from your clothing. Bonus!

Notes: You can buy washing soda and borax in bulk online in most countries. You'll save a lot of money and packaging doing it this way.

WASHING SOAKER/WHITENER

Use the Brightening Substitute (page 110). Add 1 cup to a bucket of water and soak super-soiled clothes before popping them in the wash.

WOOL WASH FOR DELICATE CLOTHES

2 tablespoons Castile soap

5 drops lavender essential oil

Add the Castile soap and lavender oil to a bucket of cold water.

CLOTHING STAIN-REMOVERS

Try one of these great methods.

1. Make a paste with bicarbonate of soda (baking soda) and water, and scrub it onto vulnerable areas of whites, like shirt armpits and collars, then pop the items into a general wash.
2. Dab some eucalyptus oil onto the stain and then wash as normal.
3. Dab hydrogen peroxide (3%) on spot stains, leave for 5 minutes, then wash as normal.

YUMMY-SMELLING FABRIC SOFTENER

No more nastiness creating up to 90 per cent of your indoor air pollution, as traditional fabric softeners are estimated to do.

20–30 drops essential oil/s of your choice

540 g (1 lb 3 oz/2 cups) Epsom salts

95 g (3¼ oz/½ cup) bicarbonate of soda (baking soda)

Simply mix the essential oil/s into the Epsom salts, then mix in the bicarbonate of soda. Keep in a jar.

About halfway through a wash (or even from the beginning), add ⅓ cup of your mixture.

DRYING YOUR CLOTHES

Dryer balls are great for reducing static and cutting drying time if you use a dryer. You can either buy them or – believe it or not – make your own. Look online. First one to Instagram that, I'm sending you a free book to give to your friend of choice!

Or you can just hang your clothes on the line and let nature do the work. Choose pegs made from wood, bamboo or stainless-steel wire.

A NOTE ON DRY-CLEANING

The principal ingredient in dry-cleaning is the nasty and super toxic 'PERC' – perchloroethylene (aka tetrachloroethylene or PCE). Long-term exposure may affect health, and it's listed as a carcinogen. Perchloroethylene is a colourless, nonflammable liquid with a sweet ether-like odour. This 'multi-system toxin' can affect fertility, and the skin, eyes, nose, throat and bladder. If you can't find a green dry-cleaner near you, consider steam-cleaning your own clothes, spot-stain removing (see number 3 opposite), handwashing where possible, and deodorising by putting the item in the freezer overnight.

✳ TO DO! ✳

✓ Develop your cleaning strategy. If you're not a DIYer, check out lowtoxlife.com/book-resources. As you run out of things, choose what you're going to replace first.

✓ If you have a cleaner, talk them through the cleaning changes you're making and the replacements you want them to use. Explain that this is for their health too!

COOKWARE AND BAKEWARE

We need. We want. We deserve ... And yet when we do get it, we're no happier, no less frazzled trying to get it all done, no more fulfilled. Something's up with that, and there's no greater example of mass consumption than in the average kitchen.

I did the dreaded second drawer in the kitchen last year – is yours a jungle too? I thought it'd be impossible to extract 20 useless things from that drawer given all the essentials in there – the microplane, measuring spoons, scissors. Sure enough, though, I found the 20 I'd challenged myself to find. I put them in a bag for my cleaner, who was moving to a new flat away from her share house and so was thrilled. And you know what? I can't even remember what they were, except that there were six wooden spoons in the mix, leaving me with only three. I really don't need more than three, so what was I doing with nine? The drawer still looks like a jungle, but, you know, it is the second drawer after all.

The kitchen done right is an investment. We have the opportunity here to invest in some pieces that make it multigenerational. I know this, because my grandmother had Le Creuset pieces in the early 1970s that are now mine.

Buy better. Buy *way* less often, and let's see what can stay and what can go in our kitchen ...

WHAT'S LEAVING THE KITCHEN

· · · · · ·

✗ Aluminium pots and pans.

✗ Nonstick (PTFE-, PFOA- or PFC-coated) frying pans, saucepans, sandwich presses, toasted-sandwich makers and baking trays.

✗ Stainless-steel pans containing nickel (which can potentially leach into the food and cause problems for those with nickel allergies).

✗ Copper pans (which can raise copper levels excessively).

✗ Plastic and cheap bamboo chopping boards.

✗ Any pressure cooker, rice cooker, slow cooker or bread maker with nonstick or plastic parts.

✗ Electric kettle.

✗ Plastic utensils.

✗ Silicone for baking (save it for cold uses and freezing only).

WHAT'S JOINING YOU
IN THE KITCHEN

· · · · · ·

✓ Cast-iron pans, waffle pans and toasted-sandwich makers.

✓ Black steel or brushed metal – my favourite natural nonstick surface.

✓ Ceramic and enamel-coated cast-iron pots and pans, and you definitely need a big French casserole dish for fuss-free, low-temperature cooking.

✓ Nickel-free stainless-steel pans.

✓ Glass bakeware.

✓ Stainless-steel bakeware, such as baking sheets and muffin tins.

✓ Hardwood chopping boards.

✓ Enamel or glass stovetop kettle.

✓ Wooden and stainless-steel utensils.

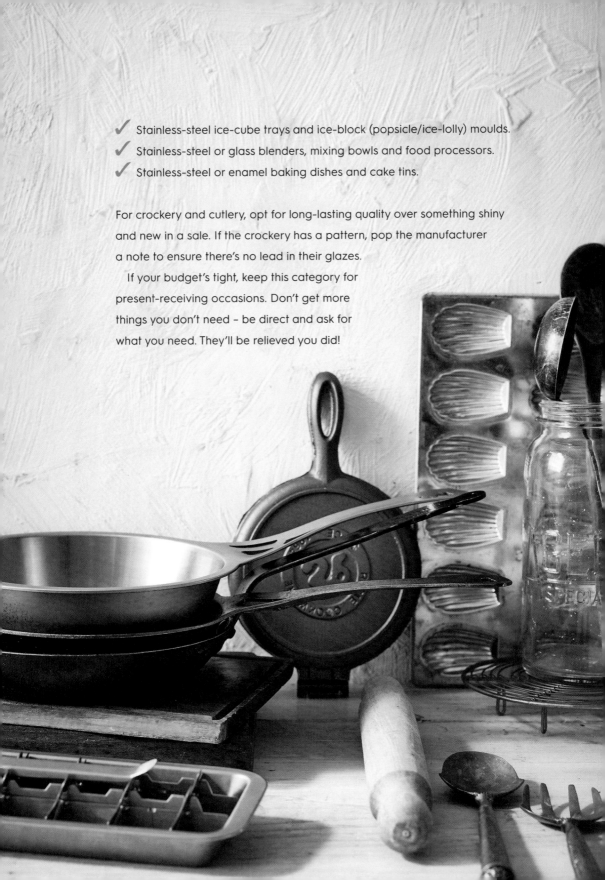

✓ Stainless-steel ice-cube trays and ice-block (popsicle/ice-lolly) moulds.

✓ Stainless-steel or glass blenders, mixing bowls and food processors.

✓ Stainless-steel or enamel baking dishes and cake tins.

For crockery and cutlery, opt for long-lasting quality over something shiny and new in a sale. If the crockery has a pattern, pop the manufacturer a note to ensure there's no lead in their glazes.

If your budget's tight, keep this category for present-receiving occasions. Don't get more things you don't need – be direct and ask for what you need. They'll be relieved you did!

HOME FRAGRANCE AND CANDLES

Have a little think for a minute about what smells good and true. A jasmine plant you walk past, fresh flowers at the market, pine cones, sea air ... Now think about the 'Pine Fresh' or 'Spring Bouquet' or 'Vanilla Crème Brûlée' fragrance claims on air fresheners, scented candles and reed fragrances. Really think about how they smell. Were you dazzled by the shiny and new?

Look at this ingredients list for a common home fragrance product. Does it fill you with thoughts of lavender fields and floral bouquets, now that you know what you know? '1,4-dichlorobenzene, terpene, di-ethyl phthalate, di-n-butyl phthalate, di-isobutyl phthalate, di-methyl phthalate, diisohexyl phthalate, galaxolide, tonalide.'

Hardly the ocean breeze 'clean-air system' we thought we were buying, eh? Let's get back to good and true. Are the very things marketed to us as 'improving our indoor air spaces' actually polluting our spaces more than anything? Wouldn't that be crazy?

CANDLES

• • • • • •

Surely, you're thinking, scented candles can't be as bad as plug-in air-fresheners. I'll give you the fact that they don't have as much packaging, but that's about it, most of the time.

Wax types are often paraffin (made from petroleum), soy (which can be GM) or palm (a deforestation disaster). The cheaper candles can also have lead in the wicks. Let the good times roll, eh?

The scents in these candles are either as bad, or use a blend of essential oils and synthetics, which means there are most likely phthalates lurking around. Even with the ones that use only essential oils, the question comes down to the origin of the wax. Can they offer you transparency? Sustainable sourcing standards? It's worth investigating with a quick email or call if it's a company whose products you've enjoyed – and giving your constructive feedback if you find the answers aren't great.

Plain beeswax candles are the best way forward if you love the flame of a candle. For fragrance options, diffusing essential oils from companies with strong sustainability practices and transparency is a brilliant way forward. You can get a diffuser and create your own blends. It's such fun to get into perfuming your home naturally, and you'll feel the difference straight away – it's like letting nature into your home, even if you live in an apartment.

SIMPLE HOME FRAGRANCE IDEAS

· · · · · ·

* **Bathroom air freshener:** Pop a few drops of essential oil on the inside of your toilet roll.

* **Long car drive spray:** Try a car freshener spray for alertness: 4 drops peppermint essential oil, 4 drops rosemary oil, 60 ml (2 fl oz/¼ cup) alcohol (e.g. vodka) and 60 ml (2 fl oz/¼ cup) water in a small spray bottle.

* **Natural air freshener 1:** Pop 60 ml (2 fl oz/¼ cup) alcohol (e.g. vodka) into a spray bottle with 125 ml (4 fl oz/½ cup) water. Add a total of 20 drops of your favourite essential oils. Spray as needed.

* **Natural air freshener 2:** Pop 45 g (1½ oz/½ cup) coffee beans in a vase with some vanilla bean powder, and sit a big beeswax candle inside.

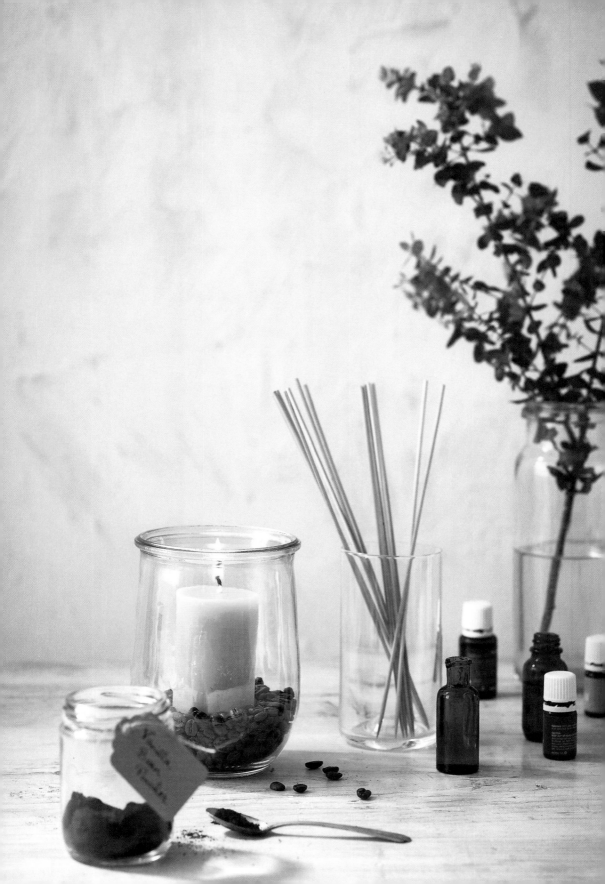

The gentle heat from the candle will bring out a beautiful, subtle vanilla bean and coffee aroma. You can also pop a baking tray of coffee beans with a ½ teaspoon vanilla powder and 3 drops cinnamon oil in a 180°C (350°F) oven for 15 minutes. It's as close as you can get to baking something extraordinary without actually baking. In fact, why don't you just bake something gorgeous? There's an idea! Nothing like the smell of something baking to lift the spirits of everyone in the house.

* **Bedroom air freshener:** For stale smelly children's bedrooms, pop a tub of bicarbonate of soda (baking soda) and 10 drops lemon oil underneath their beds. Add a few fresh drops of oil each week. They'll almost smell as sweet as the day they were born. Almost.

✳ TO DO! ✳

✓ Take the low tox challenge: Ditch all the synthetic fragrance candles and fresheners from your house. If you're not prepared to fully concede yet, that's fine. Just pop them in the garage in a box. Leave them out of your house for three weeks. Wait until you start to smell these things out and about in stores and at friends' houses. How did you go? My guess is, as with thousands before you, it will hit you like a ton of bricks just how synthetic those fragrances are.

WATER

The reality is that while most of us – thankfully – have access to better water than many less fortunate places in the world, that doesn't necessarily mean that the standards are the best they could be.

Whether or not you want to explore fluoride in the water and potential benefits or hindrances to your health (it'll take you far longer than we have space for here, but I urge you to do your research objectively and decide for yourself, taking into account the countries that do or don't fluoridate and what research they've used to come to that decision), there are other things you might want to consider removing from your tap water:

✗ chlorine and chloramine (an ammonia derivative containing chlorine)
✗ pesticide residues
✗ harmful bacteria
✗ heavy metals.

So it's a great idea to get a water filter.

You have benchtop options, whole-house options, under-sink options and shower-filter options. The shower filter is wonderful for reducing chlorine in water, and is especially great for people who tend to get red, itchy and blotchy after showers in regular town water. It can be life-changing.

Basically, in your search, you want to ensure that the filter will remove everything you want removed, and that minerals are replaced or retained in the various filtration stages.

WATER-FILTER Q&A

· · · · · ·

Ask yourself these questions to decide what type of filter you might need.

How much water do I need, and how quickly do I need it?

If you have a large family with children, and a busy life, you may need real-time filtration or an automatic reverse-osmosis system rather than a slow, small-capacity jug-type filter. If you're a couple or a small family, a counter-top or jug-type filter will be enough.

How much and what part of my water should be filtered?

If the filtered water is just for drinking and cooking, under-sink filters are the most economical. If you want clean water for your shower, you can use a shower filter. If you want all the water in your household filtered, a whole-house system is the way to go.

How much do I want to spend? If your budget is small, you can buy

a single counter-top filter or a gravity-fed terracotta or ceramic filter. If your budget is medium, a two-stage or three-stage under-sink system or a manual reverse-osmosis system are within your budget. If you can spend more, a deluxe, under-sink, automatic reverse-osmosis system or a distiller could be yours, as could the whole-house option.

Can't I just boil the water to get rid of all the bad stuff?

Unfortunately, no. It kills bacteria if well boiled, and a small amount of the chlorine will evaporate, but the rest will remain. It's better than nothing, though, if you're feeding a baby.

What if I have to swim in a chlorinated pool? Wear a generous

amount of your favourite body oil to act as a bit of a barrier when you swim.

Your health practitioner might also recommend a regular dose of vitamin C and zinc if you're in pools often.

Could I just buy my water in plastic bottles? Setting aside the fact that this is way more expensive than filtering tap water, unfortunately, from a health perspective, research shows that water is eventually contaminated, to varying degrees, by components of the plastic over time. Hot warehouses and palettes awaiting delivery in the sun can accelerate this leaching. And then there's the cost to the planet. Consider these US facts:

✳ It takes 17 million barrels of oil each year to make the bottles needed to meet the population's demand for bottled water. That's enough for 1.3 million cars for a year. This isn't counting the fuel used to transport the water to and from the factory.

✳ In 2006, the average American recycled only 23 per cent of the 50 billion water bottles they used. That's more than $1 billion worth of plastic wasted.

✳ PET plastic bottles can contain trace amounts of antimony, which in small doses can cause dizziness and depression, and in larger doses can cause nausea, vomiting and death.

Houston, we have a problem: and a big part of it is plastic water bottles!

So, get yourself a reusable stainless-steel bottle with a silicone or rubber mouthpiece, or a glass bottle with a protective cork or silicone outer, and save yourself the health risks, cost and *huge* environmental damage with every sip. That leads us perfectly from talking about water to starting to talk about plastic.

GOING LOW-PLASTIC IN A HIGH-PLASTIC WORLD

Single-use plastics and plastic in general are basically a human addiction. The average person knows that plastic is overused and wasteful, yet they just have to get that bottle of water, the takeaway coffee, the bag for their convenience.

Step one in moving forward from addictions? Admitting we have a problem. That's exactly what I had to do to reduce my plastic use. And while I'm by no means one of those admirable zero-waste gurus whose year's worth of plastic fits into one tiny jar, I'm a darn sight better than I used to be, saving thousands and thousands of single-use plastic items each year. Just me and my family. Care to join us and give it a red-hot go?

PLASTIC FACTS

Here are a few things about plastic to help you get motivated about ditching as much as you can from your day-to-day purchases:

* In 2002 alone, 5 trillion plastic bags were produced. They never fully degrade, they simply break down into microplastics, affecting wildlife and human life as we ingest them without knowing.
* BPA-free plastics may be even worse for you than those containing BPA, because alternatives like BPF might be even more harmful. There's more and more evidence coming to light on this every day.

* Some of the chemicals in plastic have been found to be obesogenic – causing you to put on weight!
* Roughly 50 per cent of the world's plastic production is used once and then thrown away. Madness!
* The amount of plastic produced in the past ten years is equal to the amount produced in the entire 20th century since plastic production began in the late 1940s.
* Throughout the world, around 1 million seabirds and 100,000 marine mammals are killed every year by plastics, either entangled and strangled or choked and starved.

REDUCING YOUR PLASTIC USE AT THE SHOPS AND AT HOME

· · · · · ·

X **Stop using plastic bags when shopping:** This means both individual plastic bags for produce and plastic bags for carting your shopping home. There's absolutely no need for three lemons to go into a single-use plastic bag that then gets packed into a single-use plastic bag. We only ever do what we do because we've been conditioned to, to the point where our brains aren't thinking any more because they don't believe they have to. In doing the work on why our plastic use needs to be drastically reduced, your brain will be able to create a new pathway and habit. Get some reusable shopping and produce bags. Don't let yourself take another plastic bag. Be strict. When you unpack the shopping, immediately place the reusable bags back in front of your front door so that you remember to take them with you. When I first imposed the bag ban, that meant wrapping shopping in my gym towel, or carrying six avocados in my handbag (I'm pretty sure people thought I was a shoplifter on the way home!). Whatever I wanted had to fit in my hands or handbag or I'd have to leave it, because I was not allowed a plastic bag full stop! I was remembering those reusable bags pretty easily after a week or two!

✓ **Buying nuts, seeds and other dried goods in bulk:** Rather than buy dried goods at the supermarket or (most) health food stores, buy them at a bulk-bin place or a co-op if you can join one in your area.

✗ **Stop buying 'halves' of fruit and veg:** Half a melon, pumpkin (squash), cauliflower, cabbage or papaya means plastic wrap. Buy them whole and get a little recipe inspiration to ensure you use them all up over the week. You could roast half your cauliflower with turmeric and olive oil, served with pomegranate and goat's curd; then blitz the other half into a purée with coconut milk and sea salt. Different textures and flavours means not getting bored!

✓ **Get reusable bags for delicate produce:** Or make your own.

✓ **Keep herbs fresh by wrapping tightly in damp tea towels:** Rather than use plastic bags. Works a treat!

✓ **Ask for a box from the store room:** This is the solution if you've forgotten your bag and you need more than you can carry. I'm waiting for the day when this stops being met with a blank stare! But truly, there's always a box lying about in the back of a shop.

✓ **Carry your own cutlery:** Keep it in a pencil case in your bag for when you do food courts and touristy days in general, where you might be handed plastic cutlery.

✓ **Buy toilet paper online:** Ditch the plastic-wrapped paper and buy loo paper online from companies that pack in card and paper. You can then use the packaging elements to wrap things and do craft.

✓ **When you have to buy in plastic, buy big bottles:** If you're not keen on soap or making your own and you really want to buy things like handwash, you can cut down on those harder-to-recycle plastics by doubling the size of what you buy. Often the container can be recycled but the little pump or lid can't, so bigger is better.

✗ **Say no to straws:** You can do it. You can lift that glass to your lips and take a sip like a plastic-saving superhero. I know you can! The issue you'll have here, though, is the bartender popping the straw in the drink on autopilot, so keep watch and cue the slow-motion 'Nooooooooo' when the straw gets picked up. Sensitive teeth? BYO steel straw.

✓ **Have your coffee at the cafe or take a reusable cup:** There are so many gorgeous reusable cup options these days, or of course the startling option of actually taking 10 minutes to sit, enjoy some slow time and have your coffee right there at the cafe. On a single trip from Sydney to LA to France back through New York and to Sydney I saved 47 new cups from being used by having my one reusable cup with me for the airports and flights alone. How's that for impact?

✓ **Choose glass over plastic where possible:** Stop buying convenient 'squeeze-tops' for products like tomato sauce, honey and mayo. Choose a glass jar or make your condiments yourself. You can grab a teaspoon and take out what you need. You don't need a squeeze bottle. They told you to, and you did it. Mute the ads and save the planet. You can reuse the glass jars for pantry items, storing stock and so on. Enter your new glass-jar addiction if it hasn't begun already ...

✓ **Jars. Jars. Jars:** I have them everywhere and use them for everything! If you're freezing leftovers in jars to avoid plastic, be sure to leave a comfortable inch at the top so the jar doesn't break when the liquid expands during freezing.

✗ **Stop using cheap ice-cube trays:** Have you been using trays that break and split every couple of years after all the bending you have to do to get the cubes out? Invest in a couple of quality stainless-steel ones. You won't regret it – they are indestructible and totally old-school!

✗ **Ditch the plastic wrap:** You can get reusable bowl covers, beeswax or hemp bowl wraps, silicone bowl covers, or just pop a plate over the bowl. It's one of those things that you just don't need to replace when you're out next time. You'll soon see you really didn't need it. I have a few tiny glass containers or jars for little things like half a lemon, opened goat's cheese and so on.

✗ Ditch the snaplock bags: Start seeing how much you can put into jars, stainless-steel containers and glass-bottomed containers, or simply wrap in reusable sandwich bags or wax-coated paper sheets. The simple act of not buying that next lot of snaplock bags will see your brain creating new ways to store things. The TV told you that snaplock bags were convenient, then your habit told you they were. Tough love is sometimes the answer. If you're having major withdrawal panics at the thought of ditching snaplocks, there are now silicone pouches, which are much hardier and reusable many times over, for years and years.

✓ Replace your plastic bathroom equipment: Use exfoliating mitts, dry brushes and washcloths made with natural fibres. Buy a sturdy metal refillable shaver handle to last you years. Ditch the plastic, PVC-rich shower curtains, where every hot shower exposes you to PVC vapours (the phthalates are back!). Either ditch the curtain altogether and let the water run into the bathroom drain, or opt for a polyester one – it at least won't have phthalates in it.

✗ Ditch the plastic floss coated in 'nonstick' Teflon: Opt for natural brands.

✗ Don't buy plastic for parties or picnics: You can get some beautiful fully biodegradable bamboo picnic and event gear these days. Or do like us, and have a cheaper set of a few things for picnics. We've had it for years.

✗ Don't buy plastic sippy cups and water bottles: Opt for glass or stainless-steel options.

ZERO PLASTIC Q&A

· · · · · ·

What can I use for kids that won't break? Enamel tableware is great for kids, as is stainless steel. In our house we're pretty big on kids being brought into our world, so we used predominantly breakables with our son from the get-go, and once he learnt (after a couple of stellar breaks) that flinging these items off the highchair was something that didn't impress Mum at all, that was that. You should, of course, be careful and always stay with your child when introducing breakable crockery.

Why can't my pantry items and water live in plastic? While heat leaching is the leading cause of plastic contamination from plastic containers, time is the next factor. A picnic spread or a drink being consumed that day aren't so much the problem as the time something spends stored in plastic. And not just the time after you buy it, the time before, too – in the factory, warehouse, truck and shop.

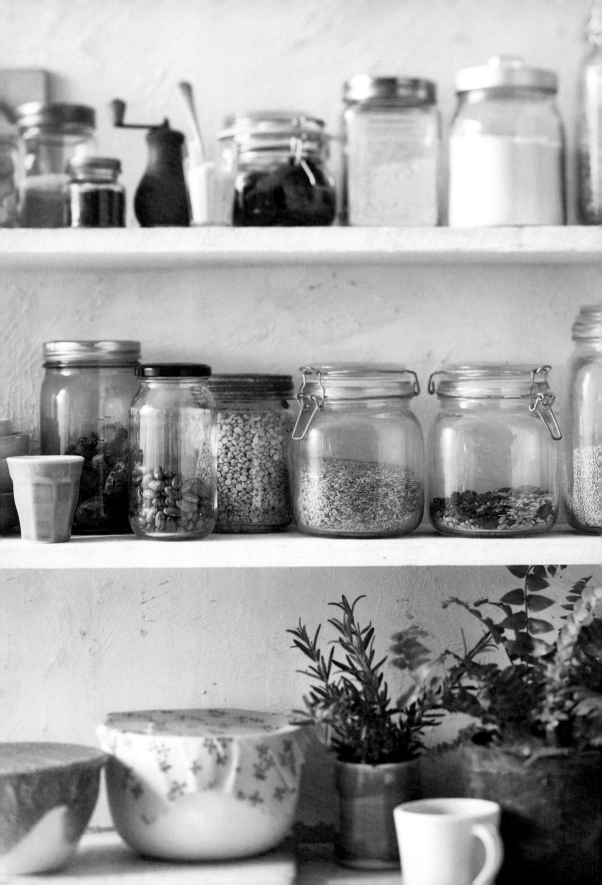

FOOD-STORAGE CONTAINERS

· · · · · ·

Here are some options to explore if you haven't already.

GLASS CONTAINERS WITH PLASTIC LIDS

These are great for freezing leftovers into portion sizes for future meals, as well as various cuts of meat. It's my favourite solution for leftovers too, because you can simply take the lid off and pop in the oven. We usually take ours to the butcher and fishmonger too, to reduce plastic usage. We forget sometimes, but I know we do our best.

Don't get stressed about a plastic lid – it's unlikely to touch the food. And if you're putting hot food in the glass container, cool the food down in the container first before putting the lid on.

GLASS JARS

Save and wash your jars from your pantry and fridge items as they run out. (Use some tea-tree oil or eucalyptus oil to remove sticky labels.) It's a good thing to have lots of different sizes. Once you start buying things in glass instead of cans, you'll find that jars accumulate. We use jars for pouring off pan juices and fats from frying to reuse (e.g. the coconut oil from frying sweet potato chips). We make double quantities of sauces and marinades, and pop the leftovers into jars for another time. If you're a bit of a neat freak, you can go for all matching ones from your local home and kitchen supply shop.

Freezer note: You must ensure you have a solid inch of room at the top when freezing liquids. Liquids expand when frozen, and cracked glass in your freezer is no fun at all! I freeze batches of homemade stock in many different-sized jars so that I can defrost it overnight in the fridge (or in the sink in winter) depending on what quantity I need the next day. Cool the liquid in the jar, lid off, in the fridge first, then put it in the freezer.

FERMENTATION JARS AND CROCKS

It's great to have a couple of bigger jars for things like fermented/cultured vegies, kombucha, kefir or beet kvass.

CANS

Cans are a minefield these days, with BPA regulations changing all the time. Honest to Goodness and Eden Organics make cans with no lining at all, and are the two safest non-BPA brands. Beware the BPA-free ones that still have a lining. While it's great that they're non-BPA, it's not so great when they're replacing BPA with BPF. For tomatoes, given their acidity, I would avoid cans altogether and opt for fresh chopped tomatoes, and passata (puréed tomatoes) or tomato paste (concentrated purée) in glass jars.

STAINLESS-STEEL OPTIONS

Stainless steel is great for kids' (and adults'!) lunchboxes. They're an investment as they're more expensive, but they don't break or get tatty like a lot of cheap plastic lunchboxes, so in the long run they save you money and landfill – and that's a wonderful thing!

WAX AND WAX-COATED WRAPS

I love hemp or beeswax bowl wraps for popping over bowls big and small or for wrapping food. Rinse with cold soapy water. Dry. Reuse. And if you use a microwave, just reheat things in bowls rather than on plates, so that you can pop a plate on top of the bowl in the microwave, instead of plastic wrap. I wince at all the wilted hot plastic wrap that touched my food and hands as I grew up. It was phthalate and BPA city!

FOOD-STORAGE TIPS

· · · · · ·

If you're stuck for the best option for particular food types, try these tips:

* **Fruit and veg:** Line your crisper drawers with a damp tea towel (dish towel), place items on top, then cover with another damp tea towel. Wash and replace the towels often.

* **Flour:** It's best to store flours, whole grains like popping corn and dry leaf herbs in the fridge or freezer. Between that and a few bay leaves in the pantry, you'll no longer have any pantry moth issues.

* **Nuts:** Nuts are susceptible to moulds and rancidity, and best kept in the fridge or freezer too if you're storing for any longer than a week or two. The freezer can also help kill any moulds they might be harbouring after being stored in bulk bins for too long.

* **Meat and fish:** Consider preparing the meat you buy in bulk with a big cook-up, and then freezing, so that you can freeze in long rectangular portioned glass containers. If you've got meatballs, burger patties and bolognese on the cards over the next month, make your meatball mix and your patty mix, then cook up a bolognese, and store them all ready to use. You'll thank me for this tip when you have abundant meals ready to go, instead of minced (ground) meat to defrost and that mountainous feeling that there's so much to do just to get dinner on the table. Next step is to remember to take big containers to the butcher, to avoid the plastic bag the meat would go into. If you have to freeze bigger cuts like roasts and shoulders, and you really want to minimise plastic use, you can remove them from the plastic, then wrap them in baking paper with either a layer of aluminium foil (not touching the meat) or elastic bands or string to hold the paper in place.

TINY BIN GOALS

The size of our bin has decreased by three-quarters in the past few years – each week our small 11-litre bin is about one-third full, down from filling a huge 50-litre bin each week.

If you're to find sustainability sustainable, slow and steady wins the race, making little changes over time. We started by composting, buying produce from the market and staples in bulk stores, and using more recyclable glass packaging. Imagine the waste we've saved from landfill in eight years!

FOOD WASTE

• • • • • •

For 35 years I was completely mindless about the fact that when vegetable matter is compacted between other materials it doesn't break down properly. Not to mention the food it could become for new plants to grow if composted and reused as fertilising gold. Or the financial waste or the waste of life if I tossed out meat or fish. Here are some scary food-waste facts:

✳ In Australia, 3.28 million tonnes of food is driven to landfill each year – that's 137 kilograms (302 pounds) each.

✳ In the United Kingdom, it's 7.3 million tonnes – 111 kilograms (245 pounds) per person – which makes it a slightly better performer than Australia.

✳ In the United States, it's estimated that 27 million tonnes – around 50 per cent of all food produced in the country – is wasted each year.

All the world's nearly 1 billion hungry people could be lifted out of malnourishment on less than a quarter of the food that's wasted in the rich countries. All of them. Isn't that shocking?

We move so fast, so disconnected from how our food is grown and produced, that we barely attach a value to it any more. It's time to slow down, connect, be grateful, waste less and make a global difference from our homes – again! Feeling powerful yet?

SEVEN SIMPLE WAYS TO SEND LESS FOOD TO LANDFILL

1 Start a fridge waste list. Write down everything you put in the bin. Make it a family challenge to reduce the number of items on your list each week, and if it's blank at the end of a week, celebrate.

2 Start a compost bin or a worm farm. Or use your local council's green bin if they provide one. We store scraps in a metal bowl on one side of our sink, and take it down to the compost bin every couple of days. Scraps from onions, carrots, leeks, herbs and celery go in a produce bag in the freezer to be used for future stock making. Citrus peel is frozen for slow cooking or roasting – it adds great flavour!

3 Don't toss odds and sods of veg. Boil them with homemade stock and a few spices or herbs, add a splash of cream or coconut cream, and blitz. 'Fridge Ends Soup' tastes delicious and is different each week. My Buy-nothing-new Curry (page 138) is super-tasty and very inexpensive.

4 Avoid topping and tailing veg. Things like cucumbers and zucchini (courgettes) really don't need it, and if you have to do it with green beans, don't cut an inch off each end, but just a tiny few millimetres!

5 Keep animal fats for reusing. Drain into a little jar and save money on butter and olive oil by frying with it the next time you're cooking.

6 Stop buying 'two for one' specials. Especially if you're a small household and/or it can't be frozen. Things on special are a food-waste trap.

7 Keep chickens – they *love* your scraps.

BUY-NOTHING-NEW CURRY

SERVES 4 ● GF ● DF ● NF ● EF (see page 197 for key)

Don't be bound by my ingredients list – truly, make this curry your own by using any limp veg that has got less and less pretty and is less and less likely to be used. For a yummy soup, add another cup of stock, remove the cinnamon stick at the end, and blend on high for a few seconds.

60 ml (2 fl oz/¼ cup) coconut oil

6 cardamom pods, bruised with the
   back of a knife

1 cinnamon stick

½ teaspoon fennel seeds

1 large onion

1 × 2.5 cm (1 inch) piece chopped ginger

2 garlic cloves

2 tablespoons your favourite curry
   powder

1 large red chilli or ½ teaspoon chilli
   flakes (optional)

4 fennel fronds

4 limp, unpretty celery stalks, cut into
   2.5 cm (1 inch) chunks

12 left-over silverbeet (Swiss chard)
   stalks, cut into 2.5 cm (1 inch) chunks

125 g (4½ oz/1 cup) ugly green beans

a few beetroot leaves (or any other
   leaves)

200 ml (7 fl oz) coconut cream

250 ml (9 fl oz/1 cup) vegetable,
   chicken or beef stock

250 ml (9 fl oz/1 cup) filtered water

125 ml (4 fl oz/½ cup) tomato passata
   (puréed tomatoes)

Heat the coconut oil with the cardamom pods, cinnamon stick and fennel seeds in a large saucepan over low–medium heat, then fry the onion for about 20 minutes, until very golden but not burnt. Add the ginger, garlic, curry powder and chilli flakes (if using), and cook for 1–2 minutes, until aromatic. Add the veg and stir until well coated with the spices. Add the remaining ingredients and stir until everything is warmed through and the vegies start to soften. Simmer for 15 minutes. Top with garnishes such as black sesame seeds, sliced spring onion (scallion), sliced chilli and coriander (cilantro) leaves, and serve as is, or with rice or quinoa or with flat bread.

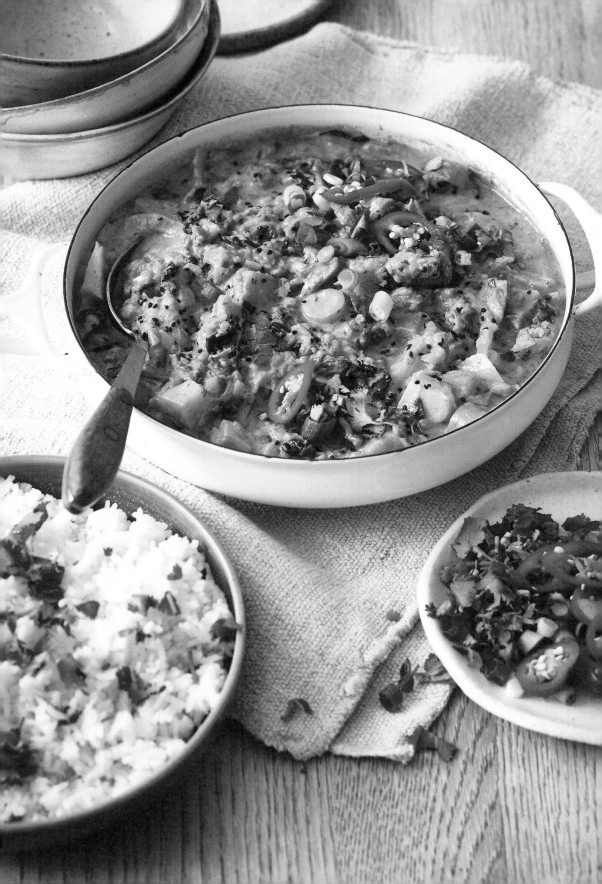

GENERAL WASTE

· · · · · ·

Then there's all the other stuff. Reduce. Reuse. Recycle. When getting rid of things, ask yourself:

* Can what I want to update or refresh in my home be reused by someone else? A charity? A friend in need? Another family (i.e. old toys, clothes, shoes)?

* Can what I want to update be sold on a community site or selling site?

* Does my local council offer any particular collection days for certain items that I might not have been aware of, such as e-waste collection or paints and oils?

* Can the item be upcycled rather than tossed? Could I use it, for example, in kids' craft, for storage in the shed, or for sorting items such as buttons, cufflinks, felt-tip pens and pencils?

BAGS FOR YOUR BINS

Do you need to line your bin any more if all offcuts are going into the compost and all fats are being stored to reuse? Otherwise, go for a tiny bin and a compostable bin liner made from potato or corn starches, checking they're from a non-GMO source.

WHY AM I BUYING THAT?

The sooner we all start asking ourselves this question, the better. If the answer is quite confronting because you feel like you need it emotionally, then have a list in your head of the top three things that fill you up emotionally, to put things back in perspective. Mine are cuddling my son and telling silly jokes, doing a Bondi to Bronte walk or even a small neighbourhood walk, and calling someone I know I'll have a passionate discussion with on a meaningful topic. And voilà – nothing bought, nothing wasted and no decision made out of 'hissy-fit type' emotion in an attempt to fill a void.

You just feel so good making a smaller footprint. It's awesome. Mindful purchases are better for us and better for the planet. What's not to love?

WASTE LESS, DISCARD WISELY

· · · · · ·

These two simple phrases are our focus here. Everything about our modern world is driving us to want more, buy more, consume more. It's so important to 'get' the part about the Low Tox Life that doesn't mean buying everything under the sun that's 'eco' just for the sake of it. Sure, there's the excitement of grabbing new essentials that you feel safe and happy to use with your new-found knowledge. But the not-so-important stuff? Well, it's just that, isn't it? Not important. Let go of the need to constantly buy things. Buy yourself time with the people you love. Buy yourself experiences instead – people who buy experiences rather than things are happier. Proven fact!

People who buy experiences rather than things are happier.

It won't necessarily be easy, but if you bear in mind these three points, you will get there:

1. **Expect failure but don't make excuses:** This is one challenge where failure is almost certain – and that's okay as long as you're giving yourself tough love when you know you've dipped into 'excuse-making' territory. Completely eliminating all plastic from your life is darn near impossible, and even the stuff you try to avoid will sometimes creep past your defences, so rather than stress about a mistake or moment of weakness, just accept it and keep trying.

2. **Do an audit and make a priority list:** Deciding to go (mostly) plastic-free can easily leave you feeling overwhelmed. So it's a good idea to start by identifying some of the bigger or more repetitive plastic inputs in your life, and work on those. Once you've established a plastic-free habit with one thing, you can move on to the next one on your list.

3 **Accept that plastic is a precious resource:** If someone in your family needs an IV drip or medication that comes in plastic packaging, appreciate it rather than feel you've failed.

Here's to peeling back the layers and lowering the plastics load and the chemicals that come along with it. This is a simplification festival. You don't need to replace all the things you might be saying goodbye to. Let it go if it's not necessary, and enjoy the space it creates in your mind and home.

✳ TO DO! ✳

✓ Write down the storage changes still to be made, and draw up a plan.

✓ Swap, sell, repurpose and upcycle the things you don't want or need.

✓ Devise a plan for your waste … maybe you could start a compost bin or worm farm, or buy truly biodegradable bin liners when you run out of what you have now.

✓ Turn your plastic reduction into a team challenge with your partner, friends or family.

MINIMISING EXPOSURE TO POLLUTANTS IN THE HOME

Your home can expose you to a wide array of toxins, from heavy metals to fungal contamination and volatile organic compounds (VOCs).

METALS

· · · · · ·

Here are some common ways we're exposed to heavy metals, and how to minimise that exposure.

1 **Lead:** This can be a component of paint on some furniture, walls and toys – especially if they're old. Check online or email the manufacturer to ensure purchases you're considering are lead-free. This applies to toys, crockery, and painted chairs and tables – especially replicas. Invest in a vacuum cleaner with a carbon HEPA filter and a motorised (turbo) head, to ensure lead-containing dust is properly removed rather than thrown into the air. Take your shoes off at the door, so you're not dragging lead dust in! If renovating an older building, be sure that you and/or your tradespeople are following correct 'lead dust' procedures when stripping back walls to repaint. Drinking water can also contain low levels of lead and other metals from pesticide residue. Best get a filter (see page 124).

2 **Cadmium:** This is found in cigarettes (and cigarette smoke). Quit smoking – it's the best thing I ever did. If you're finding it hard, work with a naturopath who's skilled in the area of withdrawal and addiction, and passionflower and L-theanine your way outa there! Hypnotherapy can work wonders, too.

3 **Mercury:** This accumulates in large fish such as swordfish and tuna, so switch to eating smaller fish such as mackerel, sardines and local small species. There's also mercury in most 'eco' lightbulbs (a sad clash between good for the environment and good for us). One local council website instructs you, if you break one of these, to put on a protective spacesuit-type thing and cut that portion of the carpet out. For real! So the old incandescent lightbulbs are sadly the best for you, health-wise, followed by LED. Or simply get your beeswax candle on! Old dental amalgam could also contain mercury, but new fillings will be fine. See a holistic dentist to decide on your best action plan.

4 **Aluminium:** This can appear in frying pans and deodorant, and of course in aluminium foil. Although not technically a *heavy* metal, it is a neurotoxin, so I strongly advise using the alternatives covered throughout this book.

DUST

• • • • • •

What is dust, really? Dust is the collective term used to describe the wide variety of organic and inorganic particles that collect in our homes. The most common things found in household dust are VOCs from electrical appliances and furniture (such as flame-retardant polybrominated diphenyl ethers, better known as PBDEs), dead skin cells (dust mite food – yummy!), mould spores, dust mites and their 'waste', pesticides (from outside via our shoes or the air), hairs, pollen, particles from our cosmetics, polychlorinated biphenyls (PCBs) from plastics, lead (see opposite) and fabric fibres (if they're synthetic fabrics, you can breathe in microplastics this way).

Sheesh. It doesn't feel the same to casually look around the room, does it?

SEVEN TIPS FOR MINIMISING HOUSEHOLD DUST AND MOULD

1 **Leave your shoes at the door:** Get a shoe rack and don't traipse all the outdoor stuff into your house. This is your best anti-dust weapon, believe it or not!

2 **Opt for wood flooring:** This is better than wall-to-wall carpets when possible, especially in bedrooms (although usually we do the opposite, right?). At the first opportunity, rip up those carpets (with masks on, of course, if you're DIYing) and get jiggy with floorboards, researching natural-finish options over high-VOC varnishes.

3 **Clean your house regularly:** Use a vacuum cleaner with a HEPA filter. If you're allergic to dust, always wear a face mask while dusting, sweeping or vacuuming.

4 **Wash all bed linens weekly:** Use hot water.

5 **Keep the humidity level below 55 per cent:** If you live in a humid or sticky climate, you may find it helpful to use a dehumidifier. We have two at home, as Sydney is quite humid! Keeping the humidity low will restrict mould growth in your home.

6 **Dust with a damp bamboo microfibre cloth:** It's best to do this with a simple dust-collecting spray – 250 ml (9 fl oz/1 cup) water, 80 ml (2½ fl oz/⅓ cup) vinegar, 1 tablespoon olive oil and 15 drops your preferred essential oil. The small amount of oils in the mix will stop dust from being displaced.

7 **Get some indoor plants.**

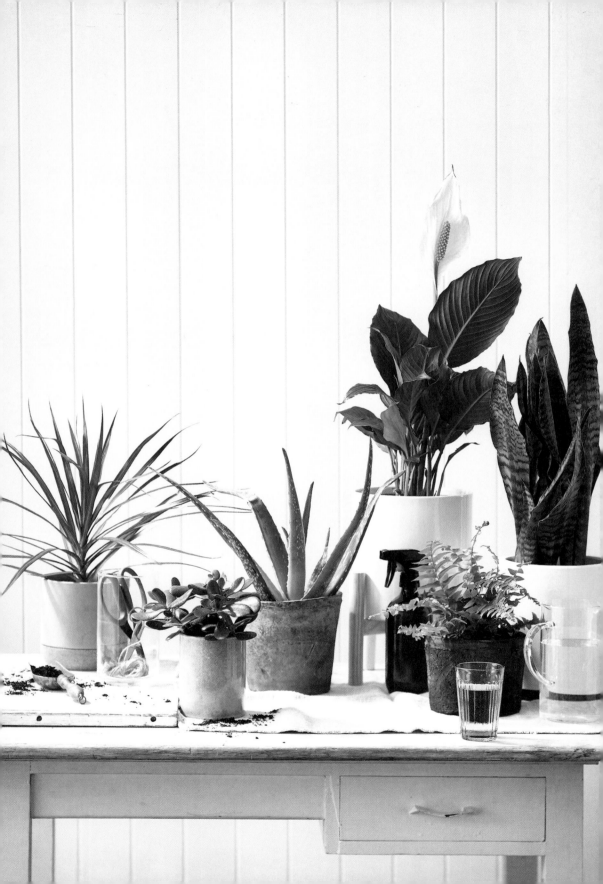

MOULD

● ● ● ● ● ●

Mould, another name for fungal growth, isn't just an unsightly or a stinky problem – it's a health risk, particularly for the 24 per cent of us who apparently don't make antibodies to its various types. The potential symptom list is long: among other things, it can affect the respiratory and nervous systems, exacerbate chronic candida, and cause fatigue, debilitating brain fogginess, wheezing, heart palpitations, histamine intolerance, respiratory infections and libido loss. If you're not getting anywhere with your health and you're experiencing endless symptoms, it's worth investigating with your health practitioner if mould is the culprit, even if you can't see or smell it - it can happen by stealth.

For deeper recurring damp problems where your walls, pipes and/or building structure have to be checked, you need to work with professionals. A building biologist is brilliant for helping you diagnose where the damp might be coming from and who to get in to remediate the mould. You may also need a builder or roofer if the issue is a leak somewhere. I highly recommend looking up a building biologist in your area to get the ball rolling. No amount of vinegar cleaning is going to help you if your building is water damaged, and it will only get more expensive to deal with over time.

If you have an allergy-prone person in the house, keep a HEPA air filter running in their bedroom. They're brilliant, and worth the extra cost.

Cross-ventilate your home when possible. Opening everything up and circulating air is great for mould minimisation (although not so great for dust minimisation when the neighbour is renovating!). If you're a ground-floor city dweller, consider installing bars and insect screens on the windows so you can open things up regularly.

AIR PURIFIERS OR FILTERS

If you're thinking about getting an air purifier or filter, make sure:

* it will deal adequately with the issue you want to address, be it heavy metals, allergens or VOCs (i.e. after a new renovation or house build).

* it filters tiny particle sizes so that it's removing mould spores. Often the cheaper ones don't do this. Given mould particle sizes are 10–30 micrometres, you want a filter that filters particles as small as 1 micrometre.

* it has the capacity to filter the room size it's going into.

* you know what needs replacing when, and how to replace the filter.

ELECTROMAGNETIC FIELD MINIMISATION

How do you feel after a day out in nature versus a day at the computer? One makes us feel far better than the other, right? So while the evidence might still be very much contested out there in science land, there's no question, with the research that has been done so far, that we should approach electromagnetic field (EMF) and electromagnetic radition (EMR) exposure with caution and smarts.

These words aren't written to alarm, simply to explore the topic, examine health effects from the research, identify common exposures and give you super-simple tips for reducing exposure in your day-to-day life.

Caution until proven safe makes a whole lot more sense to me than safe until the poop hits the fan, and oops.

According to many researchers in the field (see what I did there?), we must reduce our exposure levels to EMFs and EMR, especially in Australia and the United States, whose 'safe' limits of exposure to wireless technology are up to a million times higher than those of other countries (e.g. Austria). More than 25,000 articles have suggested caution on this subject, including one by the World Health Organization in May 2011 calling EMFs 'possibly carcinogenic', and yet at every opportunity we seem to introduce wi-fi into our lives and public spaces. Germany advises its citizens to use ethernet cabling instead of wi-fi in homes, offices and schools. France has banned wi-fi in schools. Large countries like these don't do such things on a whim – they look at the evidence and wisely proceed with caution. Caution until proven safe makes a whole lot more sense to me than safe until the poop hits the fan, and oops.

Given we're so reliant on technology, you might think it's impossible to do anything, but it's totally possible. Here are my favourite minimisation tips, inspired by multiple discussions with building biologist and PhD candidate on the subject Nicole Bijlsma:

1. Have your phone on flight mode at bedtime.

2. Use an old-fashioned clock, get rid of digital clock radios and do away with phones in the bedroom altogether.

3. If you must use an electric blanket, switch it on 15 minutes before bed, and when you get into bed, switch it off – unplugged from the wall.

4. If you iron in your bedroom, unplug from the wall after a session.

5. Switch your wi-fi router off at night for the whole house, and when it's in use, store it behind something solid so that it's not openly emitting into the room. We have ours behind a solid trunk coffee table. When a building biologist measured the difference it was quite amazing!

6. Consider an ethernet cable for your computer rather than using wi-fi.

7. If you must have a baby monitor, move it to the other side of the nursery so it's at least more than a metre from your baby's head, and have it on a voice-activated setting, so that it isn't constantly emitting a frequency.

8. Let the kids use a computer that's connected with an ethernet cable for things like researching for homework or reading and maths apps (you can buy converter plugs for laptops to accept ethernet). Allow children only to watch movies or shows that have been downloaded already, so that you can have the device in airplane mode. If they really want to watch something with the tablet, put it on a thick book or pillow so it's off their body, or rest it on a table or the carpet.

9. Make sure your bed isn't lined up against a wall where there are electrical objects on the other side, such as smart meters or fridges. If it is, just do a bedroom shuffle, and get the bed to the other side. Better still, if you have the luxury, make those bedrooms the spares, and sleep in another bedroom away from big electrics. A building biologist can assess EMF and EMR levels in your home.

10. Don't play on your phone with wi-fi enabled next to your baby's head while breastfeeding or walking with a carrier. A quick check is fine, but it's best not to use it for long periods and often. Go back to the days of either quiet meditation with the bub or trashy TV, sitting a good 3 metres (10 feet) away from the screen when breastfeeding.

See? I didn't tell you that you needed to quit Facebook. Nothing drastic. These are totally doable, right?

LOW TOX BEDROOM

A place of peace, rest, fun and ... you guessed it, potential toxicity! But you're not shocked any more, are you? You spend a massive portion of your life in this room and you're definitely worth a low tox bedroom, don't you think?

The best approach here is to ensure that as you replace things down the track, you do so with more eco-friendly, low tox options. This is an investment category, so if your budget is tight at the moment, don't panic, just think of the big picture and pop it on the longer-term goals. There's still plenty of low-cost stuff you can do to low tox your bedroom!

BED

· · · · · ·

The most important place to start is with the thing you sleep on – your bed. For the bed frame, choose solid wood finished in natural stains and waxes rather than particleboard or fibreboard, which can give off toxic formaldehyde fumes, as can lacquers.

Most mattresses have a fair bit of foam that degrades over the years. It has usually been treated with some sort of flame-retardant too, which can take up to ten years to stop emitting fumes – ugh! A quick email to the manufacturer will help you find out if that's the case.

Some mattress manufacturers also use stain-resistant chemicals that are recognised carcinogens, as well as antimony trioxide, vinylidene chloride, zinc borate, melamine, formaldehyde and decabromodiphenyl oxide. These can off-gas – release chemicals into the air. Some standard mattresses also have added substances and treatments to make them antibacterial (such as triclosan). So next time you need to swap the mattress, what should you do?

BUYING A NEW MATTRESS

The healthiest mattress is one made of natural latex or 100 per cent natural materials. Latex is naturally flame-retardant, dust-mite resistant, non-allergenic (unless your allergy is to latex), antibacterial and antifungal, while wool works as a great temperature regulator.

If you want a new mattress but your budget is tight, try this mattress upgrade. Get a great natural wool or latex mattress-topper. That's what's going to come closest to your body, so it's the best priority on a tight budget. If that's still too expensive, wait until sales time. You'll save a significant amount buying a mattress or topper when the time is right.

Pro tip: Watch for the words 'made with organic/natural latex' on the label, because that can mean as little as 1–2 per cent latex in the mattress. True story – it's a crazy world. You want a label that says '100 per cent latex/natural materials' and offers full disclosure on what those materials are. Often you'll find wool, buckwheat hull, cotton and hemp in the mix.

SHEETS AND DOONAS (DUVETS)

These are the most important things to do:

* Use natural fibres, organic if possible. If they're coloured, opt for those made with natural dyes.
* If choosing duck down, select a product with 'traceable down' to avoid supporting animal cruelty practices.
* Don't choose 'easy-iron'/'low-crease'/'anti-wrinkle' sheets, as this is a clue that they contain the chemicals necessary to achieve this finish – namely formaldehyde.

LOW TOX LIFE

* Choose organic, global organic textiles standard (GOTS)–certified cotton whenever replacing your sheets, to ensure that all stages – from cotton growth to the production of the sheets – are ethical, sustainable and supportive of farmers and factory workers. Although it's very hard to find GOTS-certified 'natural bamboo' because they're mostly blended with synthetic fibres, not all are, so shop around.

PILLOWS AND QUILTS

* While from the recycling perspective I definitely applaud a business using recycled PET for pillow or quilt fibre, I'm still not sure how I feel about it being right next to my body and breathing it in while I sleep. I'll stick to celebrating the school backpack being made from PET bottles, I think!
* Memory foams and microfibres are unfortunately either purely synthetic or blended with synthetics.
* The natural options are wool, latex or cruelty-free feather down, and some interesting bluckwheat and hemp fibres are emerging too.

A WORD ON DUCK DOWN

Animal cruelty must be explored and ensured against. It's horrible to think that a well-meaning person looking for a 'natural' bedding product might unknowingly be fuelling a super-icky industry. Live plucking is a horrible practice that still goes on today to manufacture down quilts and pillows. Be sure to use a company with what we call 'traceable down'. If the company isn't forthcoming on its website, send an email asking about traceability. People like us will effect the change if we just keep making our voices heard.

MATTRESS PROTECTORS FOR BED-WETTERS

In the bed-wetting years, the lowest tox yet effective solution is Brolly Sheets bed pads or similar products. The top layer is 100 per cent cotton, and they wash and dry easily. They also make Brolly Sheets for cots, which are a much better alternative to a plastic-backed mattress protector. Once the kiddies are out of this phase, move them to an organic cotton mattress protector. The Brolly Sheets can then be passed on to a friend or donated.

MOSQUITO NETS

We need to bring back the mozzie net. It's such a great way to keep the pests away from little sleeping humans without needing to put insect repellents on their skin every night or use those strange plug-in slow-release repellents.

EXTENDING THE LIFE OF TEXTILES

To recycle old bedding, donate pillows and sheets (and towels) to vets or pet shelters. Blankets and sheets can be donated to homeless shelters as you replace yours over time.

FIVE FREE WAYS TO TRANSFORM YOUR BEDROOM

If you have zero cash to spend on the bedroom, try these handy tips as a brilliant step towards a lower tox bedroom space.

1. Declutter it, making way for a low tox mind and good air flow.
2. Get electronics out.
3. Dust it thoroughly every week.
4. Air your mattresses and pillows in the sun, and the room by leaving the windows open with a fan blowing towards the window.
5. Air the room every day if possible.

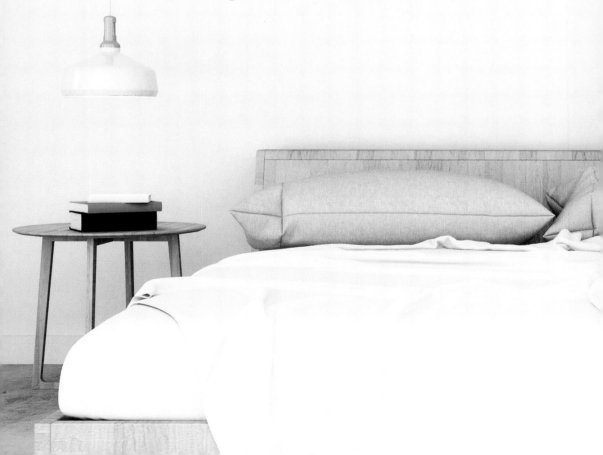

LOW TOX CLOTHES AND TEXTILES

We buy a lot of textiles in our time, through our clothes, bed linen, furniture, curtains, towels, table linen, tea towels (dish towels) ... But we're buying far too much, and it isn't always a great choice for either our health or that of the planet.

Consider that Australians buy an average of 27 kilograms of new textiles each year and then discard about 23 kilograms of that into landfill – and two-thirds of those discards are synthetic/plastic fibres that may never break down. Or that Americans collectively throw away 13 million tonnes of clothes – about 85 per cent of what they buy. You can easily see that we have a big problem, here. Between 1980 and 2014, the amount of clothing Americans bought increased by a factor of five.

Then, from an environmental perspective, consider the resources required to make synthetic textiles, as well as what's added to the textiles to produce them, dye them and ship them. Polyester demand exceeded the demand for cotton in 2002. Yep, more unnatural, human-made stuff than farm-grown stuff. In 2014, 55.2 million tonnes of polyester were used compared with 25.4 million tonnes of cotton. That growth in human-made fibres has most definitely played a part in fuelling the move towards 'fast' fashion. There's no way the cotton or wool sectors could have grown to meet that fashion demand. The pervasive use of human-made fibres is devastating because when we wash or dry our clothes, or vacuum our polyester carpets, microplastics head into the air and out into our waterways. They now show up in everything from sea salt to the tummies of wildlife, the world over.

I've shared some resources for further reading at lowtoxlife/book-resources, given we couldn't possibly cover everything about it here. Something we can start to do, though, is consider two things:

1 buying less
2 when we do buy, opting for more natural fibres where possible.

HOW TO BUY LESS

· · · · · ·

You might think that with work and all your other life commitments, it's impossible to cut down, but try these suggestions on for size.

DECIDE WHETHER YOU CAN HAVE A 'UNIFORM'

I wear only one dress in the warmer months, for example, and one in the cooler months when I speak in public – my 'speaker dress'. I wore the last one out until my husband actually had to point to the frayed edge and runaway threads and say, 'It's time. It's got to go.' I also have two outfits that I alternate wearing to meetings and more 'official stuff'. In the summer, I have six or seven dresses I wear on rotation. I have one pair of swimmers and two sarongs, which I don't replace until they wear out. I have two pairs of jeans – one light denim, one black; three T-shirts, three long-sleeved shirts and six thicker jumpers (sweaters) because I feel the cold. I wear those on rotation in the cooler months. I have three winter dresses and two coats – one light and one thick. I love each piece of clothing I own.

This is probably more than those amazing capsule wardrobes I find myself admiring, but it's manageable and still feels creative. I never have to think about what to wear, because I think in terms of 'uniforms' and, as a fashion luddite who never has felt particularly fashionable, it makes me feel like I look the part, and it lets me feel comfortable and confident in almost every situation. I truly don't worry if I'm wearing the same thing multiple times.

I couldn't care less about what people think. I'm proud to do it due to my shift in mindset and finding what's good and true over what's shiny and new. I've taken to renting dresses, too, for the odd super-fancy do, rather than buying them. You save a bucket of money and you avoid the environmental implication of having items in your wardrobe that don't get many wears.

When it comes to shoes, a UK study of 2000 women showed that the average woman owned 21 pairs including nine they never wore. We can end up buying shoes because they're a bargain or a friend encourages us, yet our instinct is towards a super-small rotation of favourites we love.

When shopping for shoes that are your essentials, ensure you focus on natural fibres or, if buying synthetics, a company that uses recycled materials – there are loads of shoe companies starting to make these shifts in their material procurement. And don't forget, there are many Imeldas out there selling excellent second-hand shoes online. They're always worth a look before buying new.

CONSIDER BUYING HALF AS MUCH OF TWICE THE QUALITY

This is probably the best way to slow down fast fashion's loss of brakes on the speed-train tracks, and also means trading up to clothes made with natural materials. With my classic black coat, for example, I spent probably 350 euros when I was in Amsterdam for a global cocktail competition final all the way back in 2006, and it's still in mint condition as I write this, at the end of 2017. Cost per wear? Worn 30 times a year, roughly, for 11 years makes it 330 times, which works out at 1.06 euros per wear. Not bad, eh? And, because I bought just one Item that trip and made it a really, really good one, I got a souvenir I love and treasure.

CONSIDER OP-SHOPPING

If you're a treasure hunter, there's treasure to be found in op shops (thrift stores) and curated second-hand stores. A good op shop will make things easy for you, with styles and size sections well differentiated, and you're doing brilliant work by extending the life of something that's already been made, while saving yourself a lot of money in the process.

CONSIDER USING ACCESSORIES

Accessories can brighten a few outfits, which means you don't need lots of bright clothes. I find that with three or four varied scarves, I'm can dress up a very limited range of simple jeans and jumpers. It must be my French genes, but I do love a good scarf!

RECONSIDER SHOPPING

Consider abandoning shopping as an option for 'something to do for fun' as a catch-up with friends. I probably lost a lot of favour just then, but think about it. I used to love shopping as a thing to do with friends, but I'd often buy things I didn't need and didn't even suit me because friends and sales assistants are, unfortunately, not always completely honest with me. And so, because everything looks 'Greaaaat on you!' you feel compelled to get it. So think about other things that are fun to do together – a beach walk, a coffee catch-up, a beautiful lunch, a cup of tea and a yummy baked treat at home. It'll be lighter on your pocket, lighter in the wardrobe, and in the long run you'll have less stuff you don't want or need.

Only shop for clothes when you specifically need something, and only solo, or with honest friends or family. My French mother is very handy for saving money, and for perfectly brutal honesty when it's required!

ETHICAL AND SUSTAINABILITY CONSIDERATIONS

• • • • • •

✳ **Avoid Teflon-coated fabrics:** True story – you often find Teflon in school, industrial or hospitality uniforms; promotional clothing; and all-weather clothing. Teflon 'breaks down' in the environment 'indefinitely' – meaning it takes so long, they've not been able to actually say after what point it's going to break down.

✳ **Avoid PVC:** Although they're often touted as 'vegan' to entice buyers, most PVCs unfortunately contain phthalates.

✳ **Avoid synthetic, human-made and petroleum-based fabrics:** At least where you can. I keep these to two pairs of gym pants, my sneakers and anything bought before I learnt of this that I can still get wear out of, for the sake of prolonging the life of my clothing to the max. If you do buy these fabrics, consider brands that use recycled PET and are thus extending the life of existing synthetics rather than encouraging the creation of new ones using petroleum.

✳ **Know your bamboo:** The issue with bamboo can be the chemicals used in processing and production. If choosing bamboo, ensure you have full transparency from the company manufacturing the products.

✳ **Choose organic cotton where possible:** If you're aiming for 100 per cent organic cotton, don't get duped when you see things like 'Made with organic cotton'. Ask, 'What else is it made with, then?' It's kind of like a processed packet of cheesy puffs that states 'Gluten-free' but has several questionable ingredients. Or a face cream 'Made with aloe vera and essential oils' that still contains synthetic fragrance as well as a bunch of other petroleum-based ingredients. 'What else is in it?' is the most powerful question you can ask in these consumer situations.

✳ **Choose GOTS-certified where possible:** This certification is the textiletopia. The farming practices have been checked out and are sound, free from pesticide, herbicide and synthetic fertiliser use. The farm workers are fairly paid. The factory workers are fairly paid. The materials are organic. There are no poisonous dyes or chemical washes used in processing or transportation. It's a label that means so much, because everything that's good and true lies behind it. You gotsta have GOTS. Dad joke, sorry – my husband will be so proud!

* **Around your home, choose natural textiles where possible:** Save up for a little longer and go for the pure-wool rug. Choose sofas you're going to love so much you wouldn't dream of replacing them anytime soon, and go for one from a company that's not using harmful flame-retardants or synthetic foams or fabrics. You can find them with the help of that wonderful thing called the internet, and more and more fabulous companies are meeting our demands and producing options for our homes that are safe for us and safe for the planet – from carpets to blinds, sheets and mattresses, and the clothes on our back. It's such an exciting thing to see this shift.

IT'S OKAY TO WEAR SOMETHING AGAIN AND AGAIN IN PUBLIC. IT'S ACTUALLY OUR RESPONSIBILITY TO DO SO.

CHAPTER FOUR

......

LOW TOX
FOOD

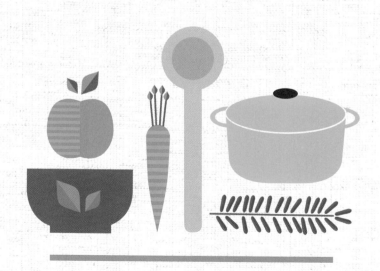

THERE'S <u>WHAT</u> IN MY AVERAGE SUPERMARKET SHOP?

Let's tuck straight in, shall we?

Consider these ingredients lists:

* Water, margarine, salt, milk solids, emulsifiers 471, antioxidants, whey powder, 304, 307B (from soy), mineral salts 339, 472, preservative 234, 202, 223, methyl cellulose – for one of the top-selling cheese-and-cracker lunchbox options in Australia

* Partially hydrogenated soybean and/or cottonseed oil, salt, natural and artificial flavours (includes: MSG, autolyzed yeast extract, disodium inosinate, disodium guanylate), spice and colouring added, soy lecithin – for a popular microwaved popcorn in the United States

* Milk chocolate (sugar, chocolate, skim milk, cocoa butter, lactose, milk fat, soy lecithin, salt, artificial flavour), sugar, cornstarch, less than 1% corn syrup, dextrin, colouring (includes Blue 1 Lake, Yellow 6, Red 40, Yellow 5, Blue 1, Red 40 Lake, Blue 2 Lake, Yellow 6 Lake, Blue 2), gum acacia – a global bestselling chocolate snack.

How did we get here? It's quite frightening, really, isn't it? Why does it all have to be this complicated? How was it ever a good idea? Was it profit-driven? Was it globalisation? Was it because we became too busy to notice the changes? Was it because we assumed that someone in our government

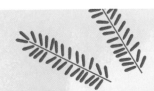

had done extensive, independent testing to ensure absolute safety? Well, it's a little sprinkle, dash and splash of all of those things, but it's time to reflect.

Here, by contrast, are the simple, real-food versions of those lists:

* Cheese – milk, cultures, rennet, salt; with crackers – flour, water, salt
* Popcorn kernels, olive oil, salt, a sprinkling of dried spices
* Cocoa, cocoa butter, sugar.

How far we've strayed ... And yet how simple it is to return home to Mother Nature. Enlightening, isn't it, that things have drifted so far from what our bodies understand? It comes right back to that inconvenient truth about so-called convenience. They told us we didn't have time. They told us they could do it cheaper for us, in convenient long-life packaging. They told us we were smart, modern people now, so food prep was beneath us. It was a chore we could be liberated from. But at what cost? With all this extra weirdness added in, packaged as attractive and fun, and engineered as tasty and unputdownable, so that we'd want more and more and more?

> *How far we've strayed ... And yet how simple it is to return home to Mother Nature.*

It takes the same amount of time to put real-food crackers and cheese into a little box as it would grabbing this packet from the pantry – or maybe you could save 20 seconds tops. But weigh up the cost of saving that 20 seconds: feeding our children information their body just won't understand. In their school day, when we want them to thrive and have energy and concentration, they need real, nourishing food. If we slow down our smart selves for just a minute, this is a no-brainer. It becomes almost laughable that we'd think about the processed option.

Consider the convenience of microwaving that bag of popcorn – which is Teflon-coated, by the way, for extra high tox value in every bag – sold to us as a ready-to-go option. Instead, let's heat a tablespoon of oil in a saucepan, add 60 g (2 oz/¼ cup) corn kernels and put the lid on. Pop, pop, pop for 2–3 minutes, and a drizzle of olive oil and some sea salt to finish. Woah, they really got us there, didn't they? I remember, after years of popcorn bags in the microwave, being so shocked by the fact that I, Alexx Stuart, aged 32, could actually just pop my own right there in my saucepan. I was a genius! And a fool.

We've come to a place and time where food-like products, with their fake colours and flavours, are promoted freely as a great way to either take a break, treat our children or share special moments with friends. Meanwhile, we see farmers who sell their raw milk from pasture-fed cows going to prison and losing their farms … I'm perplexed. I'm sad. It's so crazy, and our sense of what's right and normal has been so horribly misplaced. Why aren't those who include extensively researched harmful ingredients in packaged foods fined? Where is the police siren for them?

So let's take a look at what's real and what's not so real, and then go on to think about organics, budgets and from-scratch-cooking hacks.

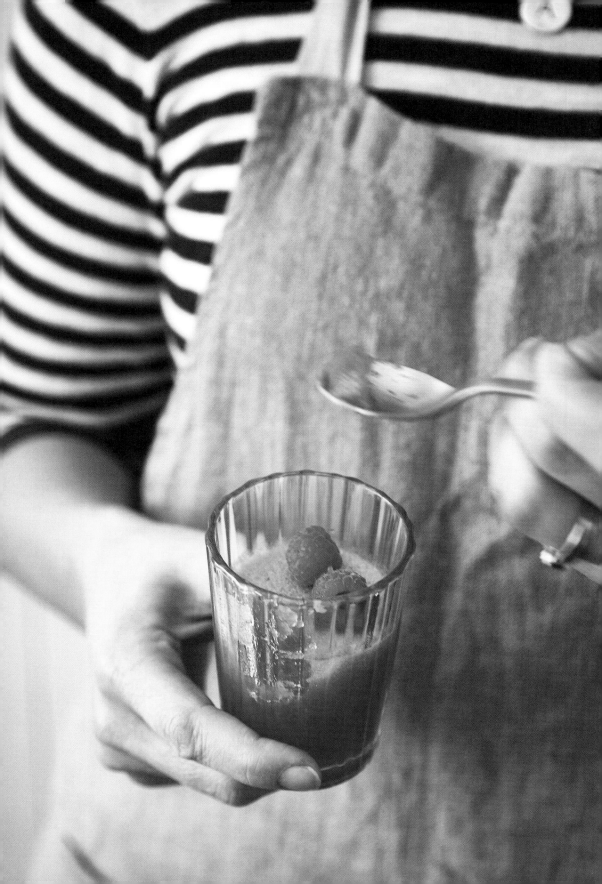

WHAT'S REAL FOOD?

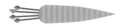

I think we should stop arguing about food and build from a foundation of simple and real. This list might help you leave standard supermarket packets and promises behind.

Think of a scale with products at one end and produce at the other, and try to move the needle towards the produce end.

✓ **Fresh vegies, herbs and seasonal fruits**

✓ **Olives**

✓ **Meat:** organic, grass-fed, pasture-raised and ethical where possible

✓ **Eggs:** organic and free-range

✓ **Gelatine:** from pure, grass-fed, pasture-raised sources

✓ **Fish and seafood:** smaller fish (to avoid bioaccumulation of mercury), responsibly caught as locally as possible in sustainably managed fisheries

✓ **Sustainable tinned fish:** either in brine or in 100 per cent olive oil; avoid options in refined vegetable oil

✓ **Fresh cheeses:** such as goat's curd, haloumi, feta, cottage cheese, quark

✓ **Aged unprocessed cheeses**

✓ **Whole milk and yoghurt:** if they agree with you

✓ **Nuts, fresh or in house-made nut milks and nut butter:** small amounts – think how hard they are to extract without all the tools of today. A handful here and there or a splash of nut milk in your tea is perfect!

✓ **Seeds:** pepitas (pumpkin seeds), sunflower seeds, hemp seeds, linseeds (flaxseeds), chia seed

✓ **Grains:** properly prepared and whole, and traditional breads and pasta from those grains, such as sourdough bread or handmade ravioli. If you have inflammation, or any gut or neurological issues, your health practitioner may suggest reducing or omitting grains from your diet.

✓ **Unrefined sugars:** from pure sources and depending on your health. If you're a diabetic, insulin-resistant or battling candida, you might need to restrict these. Discuss with your health practitioner.

✓ **Quinoa and buckwheat:** Buckwheat is best soaked and then gently dried in a low oven for optimal digestion.

✓ **Healthy fats for cooking:** butter, ghee, coconut oil, organic grass-fed tallow (beef fat), organic pork lard, duck/goose fat and olive oil

✓ **Healthy fats to eat raw:** olive oil, cold-pressed flaxseed oil, macadamia oil, avocado oil, coconut oil, hemp oil, sesame oil

✓ **Coconut:** fresh baby coconuts, or desiccated, shredded or aged coconut

✓ **Legumes:** properly prepared. Soak for 12 hours in water plus a splash of something acidic (such as apple cider vinegar), then drain, rinse and boil until tender.

✓ **Fresh vegie juices, kefir water, kombucha, homemade iced tea, smoothies, herbal teas, dandelion tea, black organic tea, organic coffee and Swiss-water-process decaffeinated coffee**

✓ **Spices and dried herbs**

✓ **Certain soy products:** tempeh, organic tofu, natto, tamari. *Must* be organic-certified to avoid GMO food trap.

✓ **Raw cacao powder or Dutch-processed unsweetened cocoa powder**

✓ **Sea vegetables:** such as dulse flakes, arame, kombu, wakame, kelp. We call dulse flakes 'purple sprinkles', and they're a special condiment and 'topper' for us.

✓ **Traditionally made vinegars:** such as apple cider vinegar with a 'mother'.

✓ **Superfoods:** maca powder, acai berries, green powder blends from pure sources, goji berries, lucuma powder, bee pollen.

WHAT'S NOT REAL FOOD?

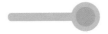

Again, this isn't about absolutes or something to stress about. Unless you're allergic, the odd thing from this list – say, at a school morning tea when you just want milk in your tea but there's only UHT – won't kill you. Don't sweat it. It's more about not making these staples in your shopping basket.

I feel deeply that the culture of breeding a sense of failure if you eat a cake with white sugar in it at Christmas isn't healthy. What sits right with me, and what I've seen become a sustainable long-term change for thousands of families in the low tox community, is focusing our best efforts on our daily choices within our budgetary and time constraints, chipping away and incorporating more and more of the good stuff over time, and just not worrying when it's out of our hands.

And on that note, here's what we want to avoid most of the time.

✗ **Petroleum-derived additives**
Most significantly found in colours. Studies have demonstrated that colours affect hyperactivity in children.

✗ **Genetically modified ingredients:** GMO corn, soy, canola, cottonseed, sugar beets. These present an ethical issue because currently companies alter the genetic make-up of a seed, sell that seed to farmers and then don't allow the farmers to save seed for the following year, instead making them buy fresh ones each year from the company. They also have to buy that company's herbicide to use in conjunction with the seeds. Genius business plan, but residues from said herbicide have been shown to cause harm.

✗ Refined and fortified breakfast cereals: If we're going to eat breakfast cereals, it's best we make them ourselves, from properly prepared grains – oats soaked overnight and cooked the following morning, for example. And don't think you need to eat commercial breakfast cereals to get certain nutrients. It's thought that up to 60 per cent of us have a gene mutation that means our processing of folic acid into active folate is either mildly or significantly impaired. Sourcing bioavailable supplementation or, even better, consulting a nutritionist to optimise your food intake and ensure adequate nutrient consumption and absorption is a priceless investment in your health.

✗ Refined flours: especially bleached and fortified with synthetic vitamins.

✗ White sugar: Apart from the odd party at Christmas, or birthday cake, this won't be living in your day-to-day pantry.

✗ Artificial preservatives: preservatives 220–228 (often preceded by 'E'). These are known to affect sensitive people in a number of ways, ranging from hives to dermatitis, asthmatic reactions, abdominal pain and diarrhoea.

✗ Artificial flavours: unspecified origin for 'natural flavour'

✗ Artificial colours: whether derived from petroleum, GMOs or palm oil.

✗ MSG: and its many glutamate cousins, such as yeast extract or hydrolysed wheat protein. These have been shown to suppress female reproductive function in rats.

✗ Artificial sweeteners: Studies show that consumers of artificial sweeteners are at greater risk of obesity over time, and that long-term use might damage kidney function.

✗ Highly processed 'healthy sweeteners': xylitol from GMO sources, white stevia crystals.

✗ **Long-life (UHT) milks:** nut, soy, rice, oat or cow's milk. These UHT versions of milks not only have significantly depleted nutrients compared to fresh forms, given the ultra heat treatment they receive, but the lining of the long-life cartons is PET plastic, and long-term plastic food storage is not the best for our health, being disruptive to our old friend the endocrine system.

✗ **Vegetable oils:** canola oil, sunflower, grapeseed, cottonseed, soybean, safflower, rapeseed. They go rancid easily and don't have the same high polyphenol levels as olive oil.

✗ **Factory-produced stock, stock cubes and gravy in packets:** These are high in glutamates and often not from traceable, ethical sources.

✗ **Soft drinks of all kinds, including slushies:** Instead of telling people to 'drink responsibly' when it comes to fizzy drinks, let's get rid of them and all their strangeness, from the colours to the flavours, synthetic vitamins, stimulants and excessive sugar. There's zero need for these. Save your money and invest in something delicious and great for you!

✗ **Processed soy:** high-heat-treated soy milk in cartons, soya sauce, soybean oil, GMO soy

✗ **Conventional 'big-brand' lollies, chips and snacks in packets:** We're moving away from these because they contain all the things we've been talking about. It's time for real treats!

✗ **Synthetic supplements with synthetic coatings or chemical additives and fillers:** Speak to your health practitioner if you're taking supplements about what the best, most naturally packaged version of that supplement is, or contact the supplement company to ask about the coatings and ingredient origins.

EATING REAL FOOD

When it comes to food, I believe that if we can do these eight basic things, we're streets ahead of where our culture is at right now, and a long way towards fixing many of the health concerns and sustainability issues facing us today:

1. Shift away from most packets and make fresh produce the cornerstone of your daily food choices.
2. Eliminate foods containing synthetic ingredients, including flavourings and preservatives, where possible.
3. Reduce your intake of excess sugars, highly processed vegetable oils and human-made salts with few minerals.
4. Cook and prepare the majority of your foods from scratch – if you made it, you know what's in it. Develop trusted sources to buy from when you have busy times.
5. Double or triple your vegetable intake. Get inspired. Try new recipes. Celebrate seasonality.
6. Reduce meat consumption and reject factory-farmed meat.
7. Be grateful for the loved ones you're sharing food with. Or if you find yourself eating alone more often than not, pick up the phone and get social. Sharing a meal with people we adore is every bit as health-giving as the things on the plate.
8. Understand that gratitude plays a huge role in developing a love of fresh food and from-scratch cooking. We're told it's beneath us, that we have no time and it's such a chore. Bollocks! It's an incredible privilege.

I found in my own learning journey that it was much easier to become a critical thinker once I could identify flaws in the system and develop a healthy level of discernment when it came to my food choices. It liberated me to make sense of things and find the truth that aligned with my values.

Exposing the cracks in the system at the grassroots level, questioning how food guidelines are created, and asking for transparency at every turn from any companies we're considering buying from, is a powerful step towards healing a broken system and letting the light back in – and preferably shining it directly on organic farming, eventually!

MY REAL FOOD MANIFESTO

• • • • • •

I think it was out of my own desire to separate the shiny and new of food land from the good and true, that I created this for World Food Day, back in 2012. I felt goosebumps as I wrote these words. It was like the old days when I was a songwriter (true story!) and sometimes words would just flow right through me and out onto the page. The success of this manifesto said so much to me about how people need and want change, and that they recognise – and are possibly just so darn relieved by – how simple the solution is!

A REAL FOOD MANIFESTO!

EAT REAL FOOD

Not packets and promises

Change ONE little thing a week

DO THE BEST YOU CAN

Teach & cook with your kids

INSIST ON ETHICAL

GROW YOUR OWN

COOK FROM THE ♥

Quit eating numb3rs

Celebrate food together

SAY A LOUD NO! TO GMO

SUPP🍎RT LOCAL FARMERS

SPREAD THE WORD!

MY REASON, SEASON, LIFETIME THEORY

• • • • • •

Whether it's based on our age, our sex, our blood group, our ancestry, our health state, a specific condition, the state of our biochemistry on any given day, our genetic expression, our hormone status, the seasons or our lifestyle, we all thrive in slightly different ways and at different times in our lives. Be open to things changing, because our bodies change and seasons change and thus our needs change along with them. How freeing is that? This was an absolute game-changer for me. This isn't a diet or fad, and you're not going to have to eat one very specific way for the rest of your life. There's no universal picture of success other than thriving, healthy people, and so my 'reason, season, lifetime' philosophy stands me – and I hope you too – in good stead.

* **A reason:** Sometimes you need to eat for a 'reason', which could be a specific healing protocol due to an illness or condition, pregnancy, recovery from surgery, detoxification, allergy or intolerance, genetic make-up, body type or constitution. These are the best situations to engage a practitioner who has trained extensively in the power and potential of certain foods in various body systems.

* **A season:** Sometimes you'll need to eat for a season in life. This reflects that slow evolution in our bodies and their nutritional needs over our lives. As we age, we outgrow certain foods and amounts of foods, and have greater requirements for others.

* **A lifetime:** Throughout life, you'll eat for a lifetime of health, and that is with well-prepared, from-scratch and from-the-heart whole food as your foundation piece. Don't worry about what happens the odd time. Be grateful you have access to whole fresh food most of the time in your blessed life, and go with the flow when you don't, making the best choice you can with what you have.

Allow yourself to be more fluid in your thinking. Allow yourself to rewrite what you thought was 'best' if something's not sitting right. Be open to what's being shared 'out there', but with the wisdom and trust that only you can ultimately know what works for you. When you think something's up, work only with a health practitioner who you feel really hears you and partners *with* you. Personalised support from a qualified practitioner will always trump someone's blog post or a celebrity protocol.

Only you can ultimately know what works for you.

People make billions of dollars from your perpetual state of feeling like you're 'not doing food right', with repeat business only coming from you continuing to feel like you're failing. I'm all for people making healthy profits, but at our expense and further plunging people into disconnectedness and confusion? No way! I've seen too many people move from fad to fad, guru to guru. It's time to focus on simple, whole foods, work out what's working best for you at this time in your life, and from there concentrate on the beautiful act of sharing food with people whose company you enjoy, and keeping your meals free from stress and attempts at perfection. Bon appétit!

IS ORGANIC IMPORTANT?

Yes, it can be, but it's not black and white. Permaculture and biodynamics need to be in the conversation mix too, as more comes to light about how the design of farms and working with nature's rhythms are critical to the farm's resilience, carbon-sequestration capability and yield. Who is the voice of the smallholder farmer wanting to produce pesticide-free produce and do it in a super-smart, high-yield-per-acre way? I feel they deserve one in a world that seems to make it harder by the day for them to wade through red tape and justify their small farm.

Are we losing out on the incredible innovation that could be uncovered with more funding to make pesticide/herbicide-free farming and regenerative farming more viable? I've stood and looked at, with my own eyes, one of the longest-standing side-by-side trials of conventional versus organic corn at the Rodale Institute in Pennsylvania, and its research suggests that organic outperforms the conventional there, so perhaps it's possible, depending on the type of crop, the type of soil and the type of support, to get the farm set-up right ... Many studies around the world show that organic yields can get almost as high as conventional ones. Is this therefore not worth exploring, given that pesticides and herbicides expose us to endocrine-disruptive chemicals, and that they wreak havoc on not just the pest they're targeting or the weed they're killing but the whole ecosystem?

And then there are the other not so black-and-white considerations. You can have 'organic'-fed chickens who live crowded in barns without access to pasture. You can have organic beef cattle that are predominantly grain-fed and not allowed antibiotics even if they're infected with something curable. I don't love that thought. Antibiotics, while absolutely overused around the world today, and especially in factory farming, can be extremely useful if we save them for when they're truly needed. So many questions. So little black and white. So many loopholes in meat and egg farms …

And so 'organic = good' and 'non-organic = bad' is far too simplistic. Something simple that works, however, is getting to know exactly how your food is produced by asking questions about its provenance then deciding whether you're cool with that or not.

It'd be nice if it were black and white, wouldn't it? If we could say, 'This is right, this is wrong, do this, don't do that,' but I find that the sooner we realise life is never that simple, the less stressed we are about decision-making when it comes to our food, working on what we can control, and going with the flow when we can't.

IS NON-GMO IMPORTANT?

• • • • • •

As a conscious, precautionary-principled eater, I believe it is. I've nothing against the exploration of genetic modification. In the medical field and in biology, there's a place for its study and use. There may even be in food one day. But here's what genetics professor Michael Antoniou has to say about the genetic-modification practices in our current food system, compared to our medical system, taken from the interview I did with him for my podcast:

> All I've done all my professional life, in all my research, has led me to know very well the strengths and weaknesses of the transgenic GM technologies.

The very first GM commodity crops that were launched were soy beans. The soy beans were engineered to withstand them being sprayed with a glyphosate-based herbicide. The soy beans were engineered with a gene from bacteria, and you can move that bacterial gene into the soy beans, and that gene will switch on, and now when you spray the soy beans the plant will stay alive, but all the weeds around it will die.

And at face value, that may sound amazing. It certainly could help the farmer, you could say. But the problem is that the technology is not precise and ignores fundamental concepts of how genes work. We know that no gene works in isolation – genes work in highly complex, integrated networks, which is why there's an obsession with safety that a given gene medicine has to go through before a clinical trial, let alone being prescribable in our medical work with gene technologies.

The same obsession with safety is not afforded to the gene technology work that becomes our food. They treat genes as isolated units of information that can be moved between organisms with total predictability, when the truth is that every gene is working within a given context within a given organism, and that when you take it out of context and move it into a completely new one, there will be consequences ... This gene will be part of a different network ... It runs the risk of disrupting one or many gene functions and ... the biochemistry, and if you disrupt the biochemistry of the plant, you run the risk of producing novel toxins, disturbed nutritional value and so on.

In one study ... we compared the composition of a GM corn with a near-identical non-GM variety, and ... there were marked differences in the core metabolite profile and the spectrum of proteins in the two crops. Our results clearly pointed the finger at the GM transformation process being at the basis of these major changes in composition. We've seen it first hand in my lab.

SO, HOW TO UPGRADE YOUR PRODUCE?

· · · · · ·

Upgrading can be easy if you take things slow and approach this transition with curiosity rather than a deprivation mindset.

1. **Grow your own:** Whether it's a few herbs or a full vegie patch, the savings are enormous. Learn the pest-fighting tips of organic gardening and reap the rewards of a tasty little crop. Maybe, if you don't have the space, someone in your family or a friend does, and you can work with them to make it happen. Kids love gardening too, and it's an awesome way to get them interested in eating vegies and enjoying nature.

2. **Shop at growers' markets:** Buying direct from farmers and butchers will often save you plenty. And my local market is a big, beautiful dose of 'how life ought to be' pills.

3. **Buy in bulk:** If it's something you use a lot and the organic version is pricey, you can save a lot by buying big on items that don't spoil or that you can freeze.

4. **Shop in co-ops:** So many co-ops are popping up all over the place, and you can save so much by shopping there. It's also wonderful that you have to bring your own jars and tubs, so the packaging is minimised and we save the world from a few more bits of plastic – always a good thing!

5. **Buy the most nutrient-dense version:** Replace table salt with mineral-rich salt, margarine or 'spreadable' butter with real block butter, pale iceberg lettuce with a darker leafy green. All of these tiny swaps mean increased nutrients and greater satiety between meals, which again means saving on the snack front. Find other cool stuff to 'fill you up' between meals – a walk, a phone call to a good friend, a TED talk online.

6. **Switch the top three items in your weekly shop to organic:** This simple move is a quick win that can make a big impact.

7 **Plan your meals:** People throw out so much food it's crazy. Put a value on that waste and plan better to minimise it, then inject that capital back into your organic food budget. Do the maths: if we're wasting 20–30 per cent of our weekly food, and organic food is about the same percentage more expensive than conventional, simply by minimising waste you could make going organic cost-neutral.

If you replaced all the cereals, snack packets, soft drinks and frozen meals in your pantry with organic versions of them, your shopping bill would go through the roof. This is a mistake we can all make when starting out. The packaged organics are very expensive for the most part.

The trick is to realise you don't need a lot of that stuff in the first place. Make a real breakfast of nutrient-dense eggs, left-over meatballs in broth with vegies, or a voluptuous smoothie packed with goodness, and you won't need the costly snacks between meals.

Use the money you would have spent on the snacks once upon a time to 'fund' the upgrade in nutrient-density and better-quality produce for your meals instead. Growing kids will often need a couple of snacks in the day, but they certainly still don't need processed foods. Give them a meatball. Give them carrot sticks dipped in homemade mayo or a smashed avocado. Make popcorn together and top it with butter, ghee or macadamia oil. You'll never fill the hunger void with processed starchy snacks, but you can sure as heck spend a lot of money trying to!

PRIORITIES YOU CAN WORK ON RIGHT NOW

It's possible to achieve a happy medium by being informed about which ingredients are the most heavily sprayed (grapes, zucchini, leafy greens, berries and stone fruits), then buying organic versions of those as much as possible. The Environmental Working Group (EWG), for example, publishes the Dirty Dozen each year to help people prioritise their organic purchases.

DOES WASHING FRUIT AND VEG REDUCE PESTICIDE RESIDUES?

Yes! Produce over packets is always best, whether sprayed or not. Washing won't remove everything, but it will help. Here are my top alternatives:

* Give them a simple little vinegar and water bath – 500 ml (17 fl oz/ 2 cups) white vinegar, 2 litres (68 fl oz/8 cups) water – for 15 minutes.
* Spray them with vinegar and leave for 2 minutes, then scrub them well under the tap with a scouring sponge. This is especially great for waxed apples and citrus, to get under the wax and ditch the spray often trapped underneath it. Spray more delicate things like berries with vinegar spray too, then rinse gently.
* Peel them if they have skin.

Also bear in mind that buying snap frozen isn't a disaster. If it's hard to get fresh produce or you're short on time and you want a few freezer emergencies, frozen vegies are often nutritionally denser than fresh vegies that have travelled the country for a couple of weeks and sat in your fridge. So don't fear the frozen stuff. Spray these with vinegar and rinse too.

ORGANIC CHALLENGE: CHANGE THREE THINGS THIS MONTH

Identify the top-three high-volume on-rotation items in your fridge or pantry and change them to organic, biodynamic or pesticide-free options straight away. That you can do easily. That could happen quickly. A quick win. A feeling you're getting somewhere. We all need that when we're striving to do things better.

COOKING MORE WITHOUT LOSING TIME

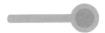

Now that you're cooking from scratch more, here's how you can maximise your time and output so that it feels effortless and doable.

Try these simple tips:

* If you're making a stew, pastry, soup, bolognese, braise, roast, bake, lasagna, compote or biscuit (cookie) dough, *never*, I repeat *never*, make enough for only one sitting. Aim to make a double batch, or enough for a snack later, or at least enough to use for lunches the next day.

* Cook more rice, beans, lentils or mash than you need. These are easy things to 'soupify' the next day by adding a few different new ingredients to create a whole new meal. They freeze well too.

* If the oven is empty while you've got dinner on the go on the stovetop or you're making a salad, roast some vegies for the next night now!

* Get good at your repertoire. I know what I'm like cooking a recipe with a new technique the first time – I read, re-read, and take a hundred steps more than needed back and forth in the kitchen. Allow yourself the time to get good at something. Asian food was my big hurdle, but now there are a couple of dishes I can do with my eyes closed because I've made them plenty of times. Master a couple of different techniques or spice ratios, so that they're committed to memory. Confidence means efficiency in the kitchen.

* Never chop a lone onion or leek. If you're anything like me, there's a psych-up to get started on making dinner – the big initial 'chop'. Chop

five or six onions and other common vegies, popping the extras in a jar or Pyrex container and freezing them so that at the drop of a hat you've got them to pop in the pan. No need to thaw them – while they soften, assemble everything else.

* Do like on TV! Get all your bits ready and chopped for adding effortlessly. A clear and organised workspace mirrors a clear and organised head when it comes to cooking.

* Make use of time pockets. While the kettle's boiling for your herbal tea at night, pop some almonds in a bowl of filtered water with a teaspoon of salt to get their overnight soaking under way. The same goes for the morning when the kettle's on again - strain the almonds and pop them in a 75°C (165°F) oven or in the dehydrator for the rest of the day – activated nuts for 3 minutes' work.

* Plan your menus for the week, and group steps and ingredients so that you only have to prep them once. Why cut carrots three times in one week? Why make a pesto or a mash twice? Why cut five onions on five different nights? Menu planning gives you the ability to attack your week of food with military precision. It makes you think realistically about what's achievable, which nights you're not going to have any time, and so on.

* Know your braises and stews. People always marvel at my set-and-forget Choose-your-own-adventure Lamb Shoulder (page 216) or my Mauritian Chicken Fricassee (page 200), but un-rightly so! They don't take hours, they take literally 5–10 minutes max. A few steps at the beginning, and then popped into a low oven while you head off to work, so they can simmer away all day – perfect!

* Learn to make awesome stock! Homemade stocks and broths are packed with minerals and nutrients, and offer great immune system support. They're also the secret to making your quick sauces taste like they've been simmering for days. Save your bones from previous meals in the freezer so you don't have to buy new bones to make stock.

FOOD

* Join or start a cooking circle and smash the week's main meals in an afternoon with friends in the biggest of all your kitchens. Everyone prepares one huge batch of something and everyone takes a family portion of each home. All your meals done for the next few days in one afternoon of catching up with friends? Genius.

* Outsource! We're only human ... There's only so much a busy person or parent can do. It pays to outsource sometimes. If you have a cleaner, maybe they can cook for you on the day they're cleaning your house (but be sure to pay them plenty more!). There are fabulous 'real food' options popping up everywhere for ordering. When outsourcing, make sure you ask if the meat comes from grass-fed animals or consider a vegetarian meal. I eat vegetarian at airports, canteens or office parties of clients. No one wins with intensively farmed animals, so if I don't know where it's from, I'm having vego that day. Outsourcing good cooking isn't failure – it's a strategy for those hectic weeks when you need back-up! I love to cook, so I don't outsource often, but when I do, I do like it to feel as if it were at least home-cooked by someone who also cares about the ingredients they use.

CUTTING CORNERS WITH YOUR FOOD BUDGET

Here are my top tips for saving in your food bills, some of them recaps from earlier in this section:

* **Stop buying processed snacks in packets:** These low-nutrient, 'filler foods' leave you wanting more 30 minutes later when the sugar + salt + fat trifecta of processed food wears off. They make out it's cheap, but it costs your health and it costs you more because you're hungry for more. Clever and dodgy, they are!

* **Start adding healthy fats:** This is especially the case for rapidly growing kids. It's a great way to stave off hunger yet give them some dense nutrition and delicious flavours. I can't tell you how many of Sebastien's little friends have come for a play and proclaimed, 'I don't eat zucchini,' or, 'I don't like cauliflower.' Well, I'll tell you what, with generous butter and a little sea salt, these kids wolf down the vegies every time in the end. Adding fats means you absorb vitamins A, E, D and K from the vegetables too – *more* nutrients again.

* **Look at the way the goods are taxed:** In Australia, for example, almond *meal* attracts a 10 per cent goods and services tax, but whole almonds don't? There's 10 per cent saved on all produce instead of buying ready meals, snack packets, ground nuts, nut butters, jams, chutneys and more. Make up big batches and get that freezer into workout mode.

* **Explore cheaper meat options:** Look for a cow-share or whole-lamb option near you. The meat costs substantially less than if you buy it in pretty manicured cuts.

* **Let go of expensive muscle meats:** If you eat meat, to trade up both in terms of nutrients and farm sustainability you can opt for regenerative farm-sourced meat and embrace secondary cuts. I buy oyster blade (flat-iron steak) on the bone, which is such great value, or brisket, mince (ground meat), liver for pâté, sausages, shoulder and neck.

* **Start planning:** We waste on average one-fifth of the food we buy. That's *another* 20 per cent cost saving right there, just by getting better at planning. To stop wasting food, I suggest a 'waste list' on the fridge (see page 137) so you can start to become conscious. I'd also suggest doing up a rough meal plan. Don't be hard on yourself if plans change – just pick up the next day and jiggle it around a bit. I don't plan weekends unless I'm entertaining.

* **Use every single bit of vegetables:** I've been at friends' houses and seen them top and tail vegies by cutting an *inch* off each side! Stop the madness – that's food. Keep all your vegie scraps in a jar in the freezer to add to stock so you don't have to use 'edible' veg. Scraps are plenty for stocks.

* **Save animal fats for frying:** It's tragic that we 'drain' fat – it's good fat to use again to sauté an onion, meaning you save on the butter or olive oil or coconut oil you would have used in that step. I wince now at the memory of painstakingly soaking fat up with paper towel and binning it. Not these days!

* **Buy only in season:** I get caught out sometimes at the counter with a pricey capsicum and go, 'Whoa, okay, I didn't realise it wasn't in season.' Buying in season is less expensive and the plant is growing when it's happiest. It just makes sense – financially and nutritionally.

REDEFINING TREATS: DISCOVERY NOT DEPRIVATION

It's really common to hear parents say to their kids, 'Hey, do you want a little treat?' while holding out a bag of lollies (sweets/candy) they've brought to the park or handing out gift bags at a party. We need to take a long, hard look at what currently constitutes a treat, because things have changed. In my childhood, genetically modified foods didn't exist (I'm now 42 years old). There were far fewer chemicals in food. Treats need our attention because the adage that 'It's just a little something now and then' works fine for a boiled sweet made with sugar and fruit juice, but not for the slew of 'fake weirdness' in modern-day sweets.

> *We need to take a long, hard look at what currently constitutes a treat ...*

Let's go through a typical ingredients list. Take a grape-flavoured chew from a well-known chocolate brand: 'Corn syrup, beet sugar, palm oil, mono- and diglycerides, hydrogenated cottonseed oil, soy lecithin, salt, artificial flavour, Blue 1, Red 40.' Open your pantry: got any of these other than salt?

Wake up and smell the coffee, Mrs Bueller, this is not a treat. Shall we make a delicious, simple something that *is*? Let's!

COCOA CARAMEL CHEWS

MAKES about 30 × 2.5 cm (1 inch) square chews

I love a good four-ingredient recipe, don't you? Here's to real treats!

200 ml (7 oz) rice malt syrup

50 g (1¾ oz) salted butter

50–60 g (3¼ oz) quality unsweetened Dutch-processed cocoa powder
  or raw cacao

2 pinches vanilla bean powder (optional)

Grease a 20 × 10 cm (8 × 4 inch) baking dish or baking tin with macadamia or coconut oil.

Combine all the ingredients in a medium saucepan and warm over low-medium heat, stirring, until melted and well mixed. Let it bubble, bubble, toil and trouble for at least 8 minutes, stirring occasionally. Pour it into the prepared dish or tin. It will spread to about 5 mm (¼ inch) deep.

Leave to cool for 30 minutes at room temperature. Turn out onto unbleached baking paper and score with a knife into 2.5 cm (1 inch) squares, without cutting all the way through.

Pop in the fridge for a further 20 minutes to cool, then snap along your score lines, making sure to eat all the uneven ones yourself – you wouldn't want your guests to see uneven work! Consider it a cook's treat.

Notes: For a vanilla bean salted chocolate caramel version, sprinkle each caramel with a mix of sea salt and vanilla bean powder. Very grown-up and indulgent – perfect to serve as an after-dinner sweet when friends are around instead of a full-blown dessert.

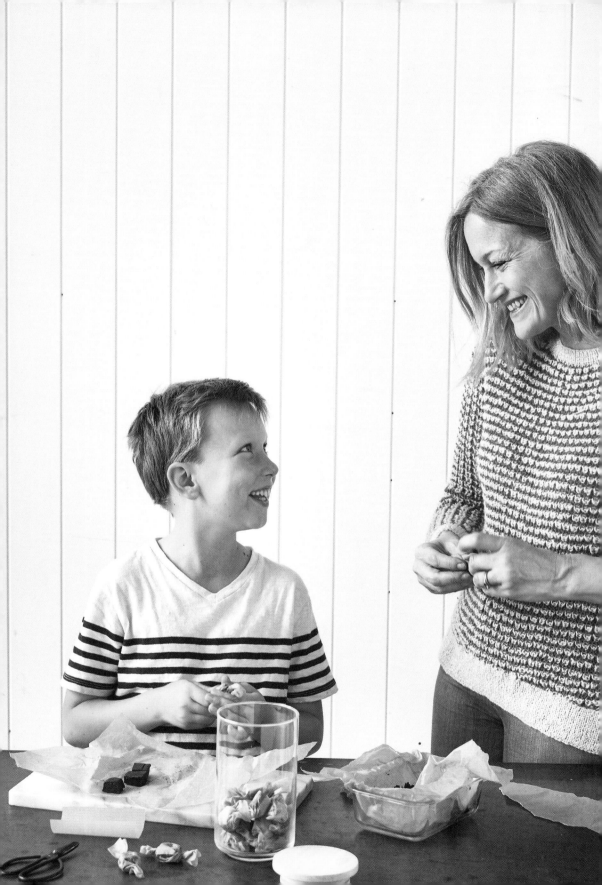

BEHIND 'TREATS' AND OTHER PROCESSED FOODS

To be free from those so-called treats and processed foods, you have to understand what's in them. So let me leave you with this thought. There's a boardroom. There are consumer insight surveys. There are calculations. There are 'crunch' mouthfeel patents – I kid you not, some breakfast cereal crunch sounds are patented. These products are made by companies that want to – and must – keep boosting their sales and share prices.

I was flagged recently by a recruitment site for a 'new product development' role with a big biscuit brand. The first KPI listed for the role was 'a focus on what is pleasurable while at the same time profitable when creating new products'. Does it matter what's in it? How do we arrive at the 'pleasure and profit' end? Don't get me wrong, there's nothing wrong with making money, but dirty money that makes us unwell? Not so cool. The way they do that is by continually finding cheap ways to manufacture weirdo products, which food scientists work hard to make addictive so that we keep coming back. Once you pop, right?

A friend of mine who was a food technologist for years was once asked to 'do whatever it takes' to shave 4 cents off the cost of a packet of mushroom-flavoured soup sachets. How horrible that behind the pretty ads about 'making things easy for us with delicious, simple solutions' is someone shaving 4 cents off a powdered mushroom soup by using a cheaper stabiliser or colouring element to reduce the need for real mushrooms.

Another food-technologist friend made an 'apricot' breakfast cereal with raisins to save money and achieve targets, then had an artificial apricot vapour sprayed into the packet before sealing, so it was 'apricotty'.

Once the food tech guys are done, a marketing team works really hard to make it look like life sucks until the moment you get to enjoy that product. It might be hard to swallow that reality right now, but it's absolutely the truth. We've been totally duped, but as soon as we realise what's truly behind these processed foods and how unnecessary they are to our happiness, life is way sweeter.

It's hard, though, because the marketing is everywhere – on TV, buses, radio – which is why you'll exhaust yourself quickly if you focus on what you *can't* have. Instead, we must see those things in a different way and support others. Bake something instead of bringing a packaged food. Let the real deliciousness speak for itself.

I became quite excited when I cracked the whole guilt–reward–deprivation circle of processed treats and realised that I just did not need any of them. This was magnified once I'd done the work to see processed food for what it really is. I didn't see an ad any more and think, 'Oh, that's exciting. I'll grab that.' I saw an ad and laughed. The fakeness is so obvious to me now, just as it is with a synthetic fragrance.

If you do the work too, you'll be jumping at the chance to sauté some greens in no time. It's a gift to the earth, and your health. And eventually – even if not straight away – it's a gift to your tastebuds, with olive oil, sea salt and goat's cheese on top!

On that note, shall we cook?

LOW TOX FEASTS

Given this isn't a cookbook as such, I thought it would be special here to share three feasts that have sentimental value for me but are also super simple and delicious to execute. I've done them to feed ten, so you could halve or double depending on the feast you're preparing for. I hope you enjoy them as much as we do. For me they're all about how beautiful it feels to prepare foods when you know your favourite people are going to come together and spend time over them.

A MAURITIAN FAMILY FEAST page 198

My mum's family is from the little island of Mauritius (I know, right? Birth lottery winner!) so I grew up with a love of all sorts of foods. In Mauritius we have the Indian influence, the African influence and the French influence, and then my part of the family adds all the things we grew up with here in Australia. When I was growing up, our neighbour on one side was Chinese and our close family friend, and there was a Vietnamese family on the other. By the age of five I'd eaten from several cultures and was proficient with chopsticks. I'm eternally grateful that I was never given a dumbed-down 'plan B' kid's meal, because I think making kids a part of the family table as soon as they're eating is essential for a happy family food experience. I hope your family loves this little look at how we come together when we're at the lunch table in Mauritius. Big bountiful lunches and simple small dinners is how we roll!

OUR STANDARD SHOW-STOPPER FEAST page 214

My husband turned 40 last year, so finally we have two adults in the house. (Okay, *chéri*, I swear that's the last time I use that terrible joke!) Since we got together 14 years ago, we've become really interested in cooking together. We had many a terribly cooked steak, burnt fritter, dry chicken and soggy frittata before we built up our confidence in the kitchen. This feast is the perfect representation of the way we cook for friends – 40 of them, in fact, for his 4.0 last year. There's simplicity yet generosity here all at the same time, and I hope you enjoy it as much as we love sharing it.

THE CARE PACKAGE FEAST page 226

I accidentally came to realise the power of a care package through friends and family members having babies. It just made sense that, rather than having me turn up with yet another jumpsuit that would fit for 2 minutes, the most important thing for a new parent would be good-quality food. In traditional cultures, for example, they know that women should be doing nothing for the first month of the baby's life, lying in bed, getting to know bub, establishing a connection and breastfeeding. Nowadays, we worship women who get their baby body back in three weeks, or get out and about days after birth. And while there's nothing wrong with bouncing back if you feel able, most of us realistically don't, and I just love what a care package can do for morale and stress levels. Keep Calm and Eat Frittata, I say …

GF = gluten-free **DF** = dairy-free **NF** = nut-free **EF** = egg-free
VEG = vegetarian (but not necessarily vegan)

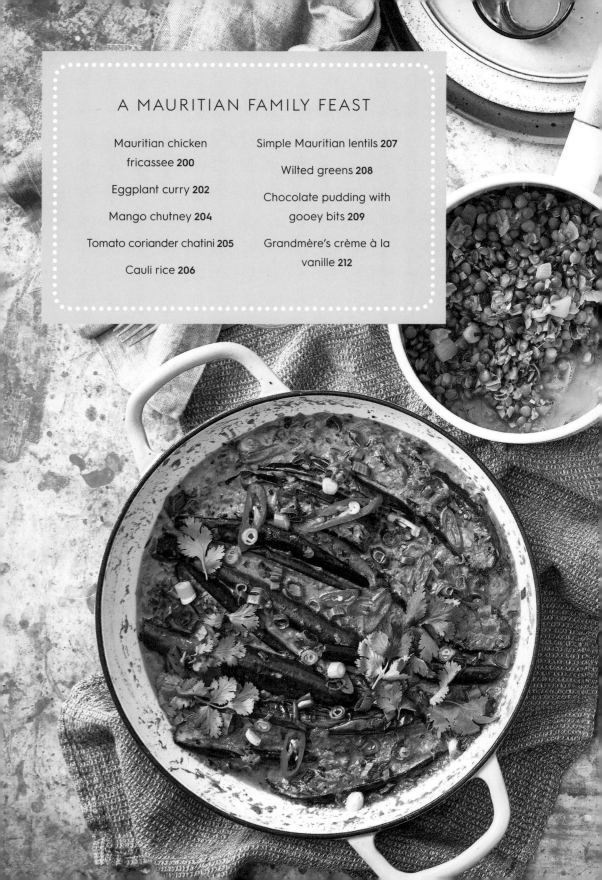

A MAURITIAN FAMILY FEAST

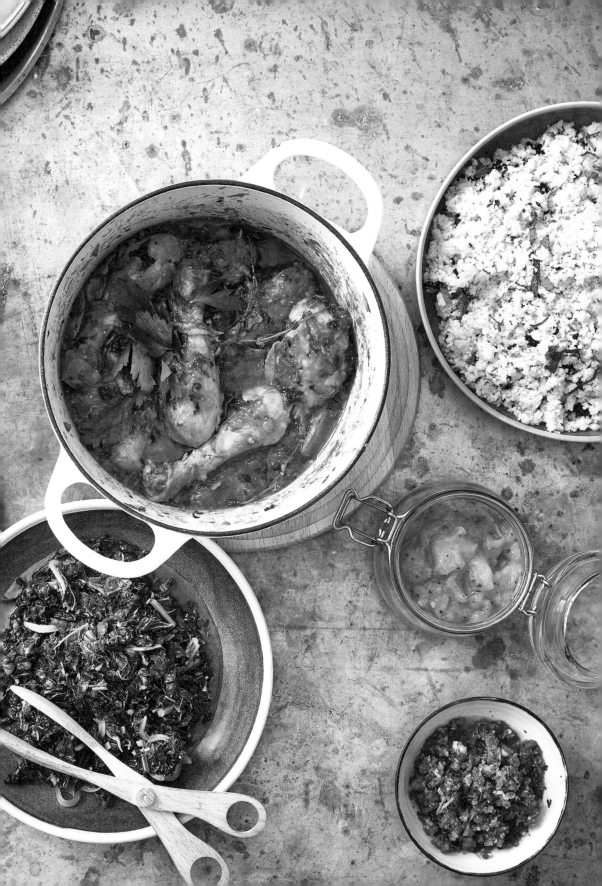

MAURITIAN CHICKEN FRICASSEE

SERVES 10 • **COOKING TIME** 3 hours (stovetop then oven) • **ACTIVE TIME** 25 minutes

SERVED Hot; *always* better the next day if you fancy prepping in advance

● GF ● DF ● NF ● EF

This Mauritian fricassee is known as the 'kids' dish' of the average lunch feast spread. It's mild, not spicy, but still totally delicious. As a big kid, this is an ultimate comfort food for me – and a taste of my childhood, as I so fortunately spent the summer by the sea every couple of years with the Mauritian side of my family.

1 tablespoon sea salt

10 chicken legs

5 chicken thighs, skin on if you can get it, halved

1 bunch parsley

60 ml (2 fl oz/¼ cup) olive oil

60 ml (2 fl oz/¼ cup) refined coconut oil (or olive oil if you have no refined coconut oil)

400 g (14 oz/2 large) red onions, halved then thinly sliced into half-rings

6 spring onions (scallions), thinly sliced, green and white parts separated

1 heaped tablespoon grated fresh ginger

1 heaped tablespoon crushed garlic

10 thyme sprigs

6 tomatoes, deseeded and roughly chopped

2 tablespoons tomato paste (concentrated purée)

125 ml (4 fl oz/½ cup) tomato passata (puréed tomatoes)

160 ml (5¼ fl oz) filtered water

2 dried chillies (optional – for grown-ups who love a bit of spice)

1 large fresh red chilli, thinly sliced, to garnish (optional)

Preheat the oven to 180°C (350°F).

Sprinkle the salt over all the chicken pieces and rub in well. Set aside a few parsley leaves as a garnish and roughly chop the rest.

Heat a flameproof enamelled cast-iron casserole pot on the stovetop over high heat. Set aside 1–2 tablespoons of the oil then heat half the remaining oil in the pot. Sear half the chicken pieces for 4–5 minutes, until the skin is browned all over. Remove the chicken and set aside in a large bowl. Repeat with the other half of the oil and the remaining chicken. (Alternatively, you can cook the chicken in two pots at once, then use one of them to make the Simple Mauritian Lentils or the Eggplant Curry. How's that for thinking, eh? It's the bartender efficiency in me coming out.)

Heat the reserved oil in the same pot over medium heat, and fry the onion and the white parts of the spring onion (set aside the green parts as a garnish, or add them now if you prefer). Add the ginger, garlic, thyme and chopped parsley, and cook for 1 minute. Return all the chicken to the pot and add the tomatoes, tomato paste, tomato passata, water and dried chilli (if using). Bring to a gentle simmer.

Put the lid on the pot and transfer to the oven for 2 hours, then remove the lid and cook for a further 30 minutes.

Remove from the oven and serve straight away, garnished with the reserved parsley leaves, the spring onion greens and the fresh chilli (if using), or save for the next day.

EGGPLANT CURRY

SERVES 10 • **COOKING TIME** 1 hour • **ACTIVE TIME** 25 minutes

SERVED Hot; *always* better the next day

● **GF** ● **DF** ● **NF** (if no nut oil) ● **EF** ● **VEG** (with vegetable stock)

If we do a lunch where there's something super mild like a fricassee, then
we'll also make something hot and punchy for contrast. This eggplant curry
is that dish in this spread. With vegetable stock it also makes a brilliant
vegetarian or vegan dinner, served with some wilted greens and quinoa
or rice. The cooking procedure might seem laborious, but it's a meditative
process of adding things bit by bit. And labours of love are always worth
it in the end, aren't they?

1 tablespoon salt, plus extra to
season

1 kg (2 lb 4 oz) Japanese eggplants
(aubergines), halved lengthways
(see note)

125 ml (4 fl oz/½ cup) coconut,
macadamia or olive oil, or ghee

1 teaspoon black mustard seeds

1 teaspoon fennel seeds

400 g (14 oz/2 large) red onions,
thinly sliced

50 g (1¾ oz) spring onions (scallions),
sliced

3 garlic cloves, crushed

1 tablespoon finely chopped fresh
ginger

1 teaspoon ground cumin

2 tablespoons your favourite masala
curry powder (see note)

10 curry leaves (fresh or dried)

1 dried chilli

30 g (1 oz/⅓ cup) desiccated coconut

1 tablespoon tomato paste
(concentrated purée)

2–3 teaspoons honey, or to taste

400 ml (14 fl oz) coconut milk

250 ml (9 fl oz/1 cup) vegetable or
chicken stock

2 large handfuls fresh coriander
(cilantro) leaves, roughly chopped

1 large fresh red chilli, thinly sliced,
to garnish (optional)

Sprinkle half the salt over the eggplant and set aside to drain in a colander for 10 minutes. Pat with a clean tea towel (dish towel) to dry well.

Heat half the oil in a large flameproof enamelled, cast-iron casserole pot or large saucepan over medium–high heat on the stovetop. Fry the eggplant for 6-7 minutes, until browned all over. Remove to a bowl and set aside. (This step is important to ensure you don't end up with disintegrated eggplant curry mush. You'll add them back in right at the end.)

Return the pan to the stovetop and heat the remaining oil over medium heat. Fry the mustard and fennel seeds for 2 minutes, then add the onion and spring onion, and cook until browned. Add the garlic, ginger, cumin, masala, curry leaves and dried chilli, and fry for a further minute or two, until the aromas are fully released. Add the desiccated coconut, and fry for another minute.

Add the tomato paste, honey, coconut milk, stock and half the coriander. Bring to the boil, then reduce the heat to low and simmer, covered, for 10 minutes. Two minutes before serving, add the eggplant and season to taste with extra salt.

Garnish with the reserved coriander and sliced chilli (if using), and serve.

Notes: You can make your own curry masala by mixing 1 teaspoon ground coriander, 2 teaspoons ground turmeric, 1 teaspoon ground cumin, 1 teaspoon ground cinnamon, ¼ teaspoon ground cardamom, ¼ teaspoon ground fenugreek and a pinch of ground cloves. Japanese eggplants are long, skinny and dark. If you can only get hold of the larger, fatter ones, cut them in half crossways and then each half into thirds lengthways.

MANGO CHUTNEY

MAKES 2 × 300–400 ml (10½–14 fl oz) jars • COOKING TIME 20 minutes • ACTIVE TIME 40 minutes
● GF ● DF ● NF ● EF ● VEG

Let me know how you go with this one – I'm totally addicted! I created it when we were in Mauritius and there were more mangoes off my aunty's tree than we knew what to do with. You'll need two sterilised 300–400 ml (10½–14 fl oz) jars.

2 tablespoons coconut oil or ghee

1 brown onion, thinly sliced

½ red onion, thinly sliced

1 × 2.5 cm (1 inch) piece fresh ginger, finely chopped

2 garlic cloves, bruised with the back of a knife and finely chopped

1 heaped teaspoon curry masala powder (see note page 203)

250 ml (9 fl oz/1 cup) apple cider vinegar

1 tablespoon maple syrup, honey or rice malt syrup

½ small green chilli or two pinches of chilli flakes (optional, but the kick is lovely!)

pinch of sea salt

1 heaped teaspoon dulse flakes (optional for a mineral boost)

4 mangoes, cut into rough 1 cm (½ inch) cubes

Heat the oil in a medium saucepan over medium–low heat and fry the onions for 5 minutes, or until soft and golden. Add the ginger and garlic, and fry for a further 1 minute. Stir in the masala and cook until fragrant. Add the remaining ingredients except the mango, stirring well, then simmer gently for 15 minutes. Stir in the mango and simmer for 5 minutes. Stir well.

Remove the saucepan from the heat and allow to cool, then pour into jars. The chutney will keep in the fridge for 1 month, or in the freezer for 6 months – so you'll have some mango out of season too.

TOMATO CORIANDER CHATINI

MAKES 600 g (1 lb 5 oz) • **ACTIVE TIME** 5 minutes

● GF ● DF ● NF ● EF ● VEG

This is so easy and fresh and delicious – it's basically a blitz in the food processor or blender and you're done! We always serve it at lunch with curries and lentils. I've added chilli because I think it's more interesting that way, but feel free to leave it out.

1 bunch coriander (cilantro), roots removed, leaves and stems well washed

600 g (1 lb 5 oz) tomatoes, deseeded and cut into cubes

50 g (1¾ oz) red onion

½ small green chilli or pinch of chilli flakes (optional)

Set aside a little of the coriander as a garnish if you like. Place all the ingredients in a blender or food processor and pulse to a chunky purée. Pop in a bowl, add the garnish (if using) and serve at your feast table.

CAULI RICE

MAKES about 900 g (2 lb/4 cups) • **SERVES** 7–10 sides as part of a feast
COOKING TIME 6 minutes • **ACTIVE TIME** 12 minutes
● GF ● DF ● NF ● EF ● VEG

Any excuse to get an extra helping of vegies into a meal! We love swapping between regular white rice and either a mix of cauli rice and cooked rice, or just cauli rice for a change. Do whatever you fancy!

1 kg (2 lb 4 oz) cauliflower
1 tablespoon ghee or olive oil
sea salt, to taste
small handful chopped mint, to garnish (optional; I like the little flavour boost)

Wash the cauliflower and pat dry with a clean tea towel (dish towel), then remove all the leaves and save those for 'end of crisper' soups and curries. Cut each head into quarters, then grate using the medium holes of a box grater, or pulse for a few times in a food processor until it's in little pieces about the size of rice grains (see note). To avoid soggy rice, I like to press the cauliflower into a clean tea towel (dish towel) before cooking, to remove any excess water.

To cook, heat the oil in a medium cast-iron frying pan or flameproof enamelled cast-iron pot, add the cauliflower rice, then toss for 4–5 minutes so it doesn't go mushy. Season with salt and garnish with mint (if using).

Note: If any of the stems are too tough to grate or process, set them aside and pop in the freezer for your next soup or curry.

SIMPLE MAURITIAN LENTILS

SERVES 10 • **SOAKING TIME** 12–24 hours • **COOKING TIME** about 1 hour • **ACTIVE TIME** 10 minutes
● GF ● DF ● NF ● EF ● VEG

You can use this easy recipe to make a gorgeous soup – just add a little curry powder and some coconut cream, and blend once cooked. But a Mauritian lunchtime feast will never be without this lentil side dish. If the curries of the day are quite spicy, the kids often have a fried egg with these lentils and rice as their lunch. Simple and always appreciated.

500 g (1 lb 2 oz) black or brown lentils

1 tablespoon lemon juice

1 tablespoon coconut oil or ghee

400 g (14 oz/2 large) red onions,
   finely chopped

1 tablespoon crushed garlic

1 tablespoon finely chopped fresh
   ginger

8 curry leaves

1 handful parsley leaves

3 thyme sprigs

about 2 litres (68 fl oz/8 cups) filtered
   water

sea salt, to taste

Cover the lentils with filtered water, stir in the lemon juice, then cover the bowl and soak overnight. (They can be soaked for up to 24 hours if you have things to do the next day, so there's no stress.)

The next day, drain and rinse the lentils. Heat the oil in a flameproof enamelled cast-iron casserole pot over medium heat and fry the onion, garlic and ginger for 4–5 minutes, until the onion is transparent. Add the lentils, curry leaves, parsley, thyme and enough water to cover the lentils. Bring to the boil, then reduce the heat to low and simmer, covered, for 1 hour or a little longer (depending on how long you soaked them). Check on them occasionally until they're tender.

Season with salt and serve with basmati rice or cauliflower rice.

WILTED GREENS

SERVES 10 • **COOKING TIME** 15 minutes • **ACTIVE TIME** 15 minutes
● GF ● DF ● NF ● EF ● VEG

In Mauritius, we use the leaves from the local pumpkin (winter squash) crop to make our green sides for curry lunch feasts. They're so delicious, and I love that the whole plant is used. A popular light dinner is a gratin of pumpkin with a little bread and a salad. Use whatever you have available in your part of the world for this. Most often I'll use a combination of cavolo nero and some Chinese green veg, but you could use regular kale, spinach, silverbeet (Swiss chard), collard greens or even rocket (arugula).

60 ml (2 fl oz/¼ cup) olive oil or ghee

1 red onion (of course)

1 teaspoon finely chopped fresh ginger

1 teaspoon finely chopped garlic

2 thyme sprigs

about 500 g (1 lb 2 oz/2 bunches) cavolo nero (lacinato kale) or other greens, roughly chopped

½ teaspoon sea salt

250 ml (9 fl oz/1 cup) filtered water

Heat the oil in a large frying pan or saucepan over medium heat and fry the onions until softened. Add the ginger, garlic and thyme, then sauté for another minute. Add the greens, salt and water, then bring to the boil. Reduce the heat to low and simmer, covered, for about 10 minutes, until the greens are soft. Serve immediately.

CHOCOLATE PUDDING WITH GOOEY BITS

SERVES 10 • **COOKING TIME** 20–30 minutes • **ACTIVE TIME** 5 minutes
● **GF** ● **NF** (if no nut oil) ● **VEG**

This is a super-forgiving pudding! I make it with a blender, but you could mix it by hand with a whisk.

4 eggs (or 3 if very large)

130–180 ml (4½–6 fl oz) rice malt
syrup, maple syrup or honey,
to taste

125 ml (4 fl oz/½ cup) melted salted
butter, macadamia oil or coconut oil

90 g (3¼ oz/⅔ cup) tapioca or
arrowroot flour (see note)

40 g (1½ oz/⅓ cup) unsweetened
Dutch-processed cocoa powder or
raw cacao

40 g (1½ oz/⅓ cup) coconut flour

2 heaped teaspoons baking powder

1 heaped teaspoon vanilla bean
powder, or 1 vanilla bean, split
lengthways and seeds scraped,
or 2 teaspoons vanilla extract

GOOEY BITS SAUCE

125 ml (4 fl oz/½ cup) melted salted
butter

80 ml (2½ fl oz/⅓ cup) rice malt syrup,
honey or maple syrup

40 g (1½ oz/⅓ cup) unsweetened
Dutch-processed cocoa powder or
raw cacao

Preheat the oven to 180°C (350°F).

To make the sauce, combine all the gooey bits ingredients in a medium saucepan over medium heat and stir until well combined. Pour the sauce into the bottom of an ovenproof pudding basin (mould).

In a blender, whisk the eggs for 5 seconds. Add the remaining pudding ingredients and blend to combine.   >>

Pour the pudding on top of the sauce. Don't panic, the gooey sauce will come up around your pudding batter, which is totally normal and even perhaps awesome. You'll see!

Bake for 20–30 minutes, until the pudding springs back when you press the edges but is still quite soft in the middle. When you test the centre with a skewer, there should still be a little pudding on it. Worst cake scenario is you get a cakier result if you take it a few minutes too far. You'll still get a bit of gooeyness from the sauce around the edges and underneath.

Serve with Grandmère's crème à la vanille.

Notes: Arrowroot flour is often preserved with E220, so check. For a denser pudding, replace the tapioca flour with 90 g (3¼ oz/⅔ cup) buckwheat flour or 70 g (2¾ oz/⅔ cup) almond meal (only if the recipe doesn't need to be nut free). If using a thermocooker, make the sauce for 2 minutes on speed 3, 100°C. There's no need to clean the bowl before whisking the eggs for 5 seconds on speed 6, then the remaining ingredients for 6 seconds on speed 5.

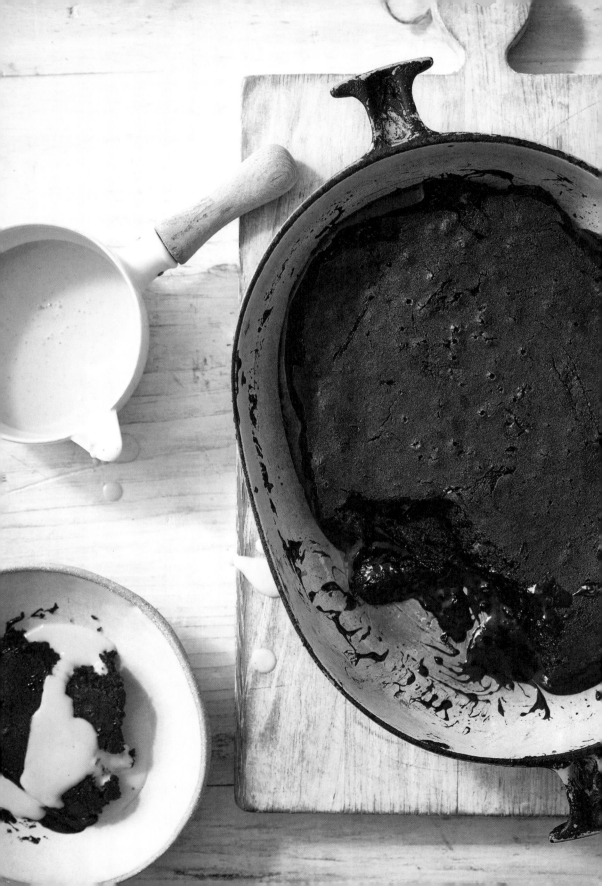

GRANDMÈRE'S CRÈME À LA VANILLE

SERVES 10 as a pudding-topper • **COOKING TIME** 15 minutes • **ACTIVE TIME** 15 minutes
● **GF** ● **DF** (with coconut milk) ● **NF** ● **VEG**

Mauritian vanilla has a taste to it. It's the kind of thing we stock up on whenever we visit, and then carefully ration until our next trip! This crème à la vanille takes me back to the days of my grandmère, who was the dessert hero of the island. No one could resist a dessert made by Thérèse, and when we were at the beach in the summer, people would oh so conveniently appear around 4 pm just to say a quick hello, secretly knowing that'd be about the time Grandmère would take a cake out of the oven for afternoon tea … And then, 'Oh, is that Thérèse's gâteau au chocolat? It'd be rude to say no.' Ha! I'm looking at you all, dear cousins.

When Grandmère's dementia started to kick in and she began burning things she'd made a thousand times, I felt a huge sense of urgency to continue her dessert-making legacy in our family. And so one summer, I lived in the kitchen with her, soaking up the wisdom. It was such a special time, and as I share this custard with you now, you have to promise me something: you will not buy that strange, fake, coloured carton stuff ever again. Making custard is magic at work. It's so fun, and once you know how, you'll love making it for your family forever more – the real stuff! While I might make Grandmère's recipes with low tox ingredients, subbing out the refined flours and sugars, I'm sure she'd understand why if she'd had the chance to learn. And no one complains when I'm around rustling up a batch these days, that's for sure!

800 ml (28 fl oz) your milk of choice
(see note)

1 vanilla bean, split lengthways and
seeds scraped, or ½ teaspoon
vanilla bean powder

6 egg yolks

100 ml (3½ fl oz) pure maple syrup or
80 ml (2½ fl oz/⅓ cup) sucanat or
rapadura sugar

1–1½ tablespoons tapioca or
arrowroot flour (see note page 210;
use more for a thicker custard)

Pour the milk into a medium saucepan and add the vanilla bean and seeds.
Place the saucepan over medium heat and watch carefully.

While the milk is heating, whisk the egg yolks with your chosen sweet stuff
and the flour in a large enough bowl to pour the milk into as well.

When the milk has just come to simmer (i.e. froths around the edges), take
it off the heat and pour a tiny bit into the egg mixture, whisking continuously,
then pour in the rest in a slow, steady stream until the two mixtures are just
incorporated (cooking with a friend or a child makes this step easy-peasy!).
Immediately pour the whole custard mixture back into the saucepan then
return to medium–low heat, stirring continuously with a wooden spoon, until
the mixture thickens enough to coat the spoon nicely, then pour into a bowl,
vanilla pod and all, to let those flavours deepen further. (Don't let it bubble –
that's too hot and it will curdle. If in doubt, take it off the heat immediately
and pour into the bowl. Runny custard is better than chunky curdled custard,
trust me! Next time try more flour.)

You're done. Pop it in the fridge to cool.

Notes: Coconut milk makes a gorgeous dairy-free version. Cow's milk is
fabulous too, but you have to watch it more closely at the end and take it off
the heat before it can split, whereas coconut milk is super stable and safe
for the debutant. These days, if I'm pressed for time I use the thermocooker
(everything in at once for 7 minutes on speed 4, 80°C/175°F), but I do find
the traditional method very therapeutic, and I still do it that way if I have the
15 minutes to spare.

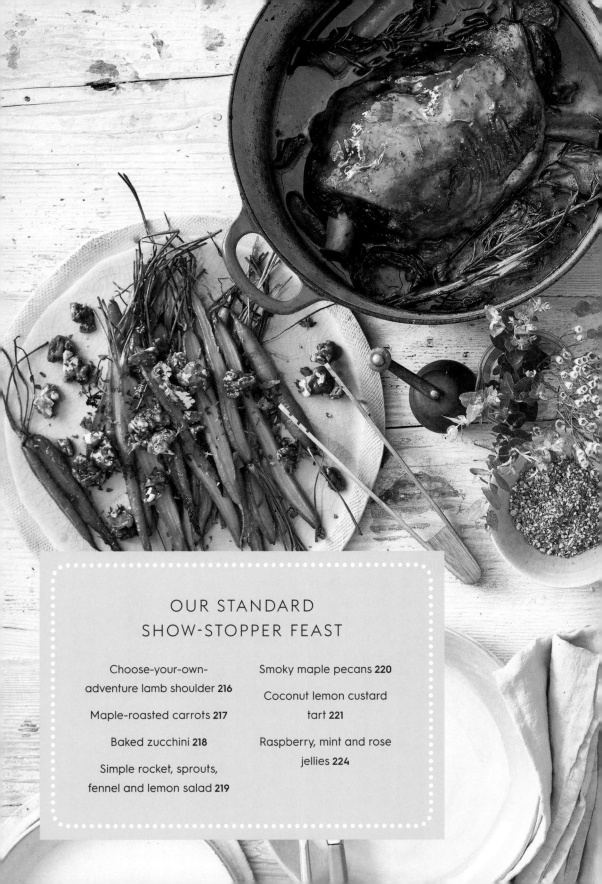

OUR STANDARD
SHOW-STOPPER FEAST

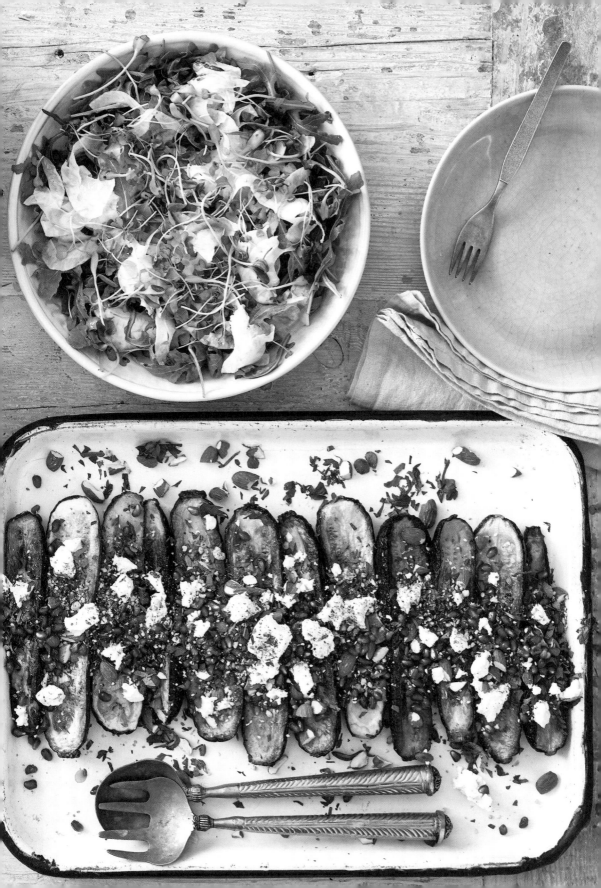

CHOOSE-YOUR-OWN-ADVENTURE LAMB SHOULDER

SERVES 6–8 with sides • **COOKING TIME** 6–12 hours • **ACTIVE TIME** 15 minutes
● GF ● NF ● EF

This is the kind of recipe you make when you want to entertain the people you love and you have zero time to do it, but would love all the same to be showered with compliments for your genius. It's only 15 minutes' active work for a taste that feels like you should have been working all day!

1 heaped teaspoon sea salt

1 large (or 2 small) lamb shoulder

2 tablespoons butter, ghee or olive oil

400 ml (14 fl oz) filtered water

2 carrots, skin on, each chopped into
    a couple of big chunks

2 celery stalks, snapped in half
    crossways

200 g (7 oz) onion, quartered

4–6 garlic cloves

1 large handful parsley leaves

FLAVOUR COMBINATION 1

4 thyme sprigs

2 bay leaves

4 rosemary sprigs

grated rind of ½ lemon

FLAVOUR COMBINATION 2

1 tablespoon ground cumin

1 teaspoon ground cinnamon

1 teaspoon paprika

1 teaspoon ground turmeric

¼ teaspoon ground black pepper

FLAVOUR COMBINATION 3

200 ml (7 fl oz) red wine

80 ml (2½ fl oz/⅓ cup) tomato
    passata (puréed tomatoes)

6 thyme sprigs

1 teaspoon tapioca or arrowroot flour
    (see note page 210)

1 heaped teaspoon herbes de
    Provence

Preheat the oven to 140°C (275°F) for cooking from midday for dinner, or 120°C (235°F) for cooking from early morning all day for dinner.

Sprinkle the salt over both sides of the lamb shoulder and rub in well.

Place a flameproof enamelled cast-iron pot large enough to take the lamb shoulder over medium–high heat and heat the butter or oil. Just as the butter gets hot, add the lamb shoulder and brown for a couple of minutes on both sides. Pour in the water, then add the carrots, celery, onion, garlic, parsley and your chosen flavouring. Put on the lid or cover with aluminium foil and cook for 6–12 hours, to match your chosen oven heat.

Fork the lamb onto plates (trust me, it's that tender!) and top with a couple of spoonfuls of the cooking juices.

MAPLE-ROASTED CARROTS

SERVES 8-10 people as a side • COOKING TIME 35 minutes • ACTIVE TIME 5 minutes
● GF ● DF ● NF ● EF ● VEG

3 bunches Dutch (whole baby) carrots, skin on, washed, dried and stems removed with a bit left at the top for a rustic look

60 ml (2 fl oz/¼ cup) olive oil

1 tablespoon finely chopped thyme

1 handful finely chopped parsley leaves

sea salt and ground black pepper, to taste

Preheat the oven to 225°C (430°F).

Lay the carrots in a single layer on a baking tray. Drizzle over the olive oil and scatter over the thyme and 1 tablespoon of the parsley. Season with salt and pepper, then toss the carrots to coat well. Bake for 30–35 minutes, until golden and lightly roasted.

Serve topped with the remaining parsley and the Smoky Maple Pecans (page 220).

BAKED ZUCCHINI

SERVES 6-8 as a side • **COOKING TIME** 20-30 minutes • **ACTIVE TIME** 5 minutes

● GF ● DF (without the labne) ● EF ● VEG

This is so easy and yet so impressive-looking! Don't be too fussed if you don't have every single topping in the recipe, either. Just use what you have and think about adding something cheesy, something crunchy, something herby and something spicy. You can serve straight from the tray, so arrange the zucchini halves neatly if you want it to look pretty.

8 zucchini (courgettes)

60 ml (2 fl oz/¼ cup) olive oil, plus extra as needed

3 tablespoons dukkah

1 handful chopped mint leaves

1 handful chopped parsley leaves

½–¾ cup labne, or fresh goat's or sheep's milk curd

80 g (2¾ oz/½ cup) almonds or other nuts, toasted at 180°C (350°F) for 15 minutes

1 pomegranate, cut in half and seeds extracted (see note)

½ lemon

sea salt and ground black pepper, to taste

Preheat the oven to 180°C (350°F).

Halve all the zucchini lengthways, leaving the ends on. Lay them out on two baking trays, cut-side up, and drizzle with the olive oil. Bake for 20-30 minutes, until they yield a little when you squeeze them gently.

Scatter over the dukkah, then the herbs, then the labne, then the almonds, then the pomegranate seeds. Squeeze over the lemon for a bit of zing, then add a final drizzle of olive oil. Grab a clean tea towel (dish towel) and wipe around the edges if it looks messy.

Notes: To extract the pomegranate seeds, bash each half with a rolling pin, cut-side down, into an empty bowl. If pomegranates aren't in season, fresh currants are a great alternative, as are a few dried cranberries.

SIMPLE ROCKET, SPROUTS, FENNEL AND LEMON SALAD

SERVES 8 as a side • **COOKING TIME** 0 • **ACTIVE TIME** 5 minutes
● **GF** ● **DF** ● **NF** (without the Smoky Maple Pecans) ● **EF** ● **VEG**

I'm pretty convinced that rocket (arugula) is my life blood. I eat it two meals a day without fail and I'm sad if where I'm travelling doesn't have it. It's the first thing I buy when I come home. There aren't many meals where a rocket salad isn't in the mix, and so of course, if you're coming for a feast to my place, you can expect to see it somewhere. Use baby English spinach if that's what you have. Rocket and sprouts are beautifully anti-inflammatory foods – they're powerful to include in your meals if you frequently have histamine reactions. Sprouts especially help you empty your histamine bucket, making you less reactive. They're little miracles!

150 g (5½ oz/3⅓ cups) rocket (arugula) leaves

1 × 150 g (5½ oz) fennel bulb, shaved thinly

1 cup sprouts of your choice (I love snow pea sprouts, lentil sprouts or mung bean sprouts)

left-over Smoky Maple Pecans (page 220), because yum! (optional)

VINAIGRETTE

120 ml (4 fl oz) extra virgin olive oil

2 tablespoons balsamic vinegar or apple cider vinegar

2 teaspoons maple syrup

2 teaspoons filtered water

1 teaspoon smooth French mustard

3 pinches of sea salt

2 pinches of ground black pepper

To make the vinaigrette, pop all the ingredients in a jar. Put the lid on. Shaky, shaky, vigorously, for 30 seconds. You're done.

Toss the salad ingredients together in a bowl. Work the vinaigrette through the salad, starting with about half the dressing. You can always add more, but an over-dressed salad is sogs-ville – not very nice!

SMOKY MAPLE PECANS

MAKES 100 g (3½ oz/1 cup) • **COOKING TIME** 15 minutes • **ACTIVE TIME** 10 minutes
● **GF** ● **DF** (with coconut oil) ● **EF** ● **VEG**

These are to die for. Some of them might even make it to being served with the carrots! You'll see what I mean when you've made them. Double the batch to have some left over for subsequent salads.

130 g (4½ oz) pecans, halved

40 g (1½ oz) salted butter (see note), or coconut oil or ghee

125 ml (4 fl oz/½ cup) rice malt syrup (see note)

SMOKY SPICES

½ teaspoon smoked paprika

¼ teaspoon chipotle powder

¼ teaspoon ground cumin

¼ teaspoon sea salt

¼ teaspoon onion powder

Preheat the oven to 200°C (400°F).

Spread the pecans on a baking tray and roast for 10–12 minutes. Halfway into the roasting time, start the rest of the prep.

Lay a sheet of unbleached baking paper (see note) on the benchtop.

Melt the butter or oil in a small heavy-based frying pan over medium heat. Add the rice malt syrup and stir until combined and bubbling. Let this mixture bubble away slowly for 7–8 minutes, or as soon as you detect a change to a deeper golden colour. Add the smoky spices, then immediately remove the pecans from the oven and toss into the caramel, stirring to coat, then pour it all onto the baking paper pronto.

Leave on the baking paper to harden as it cools. Roughly chop into smaller chunks. Serve immediately or store in an airtight container.

Notes: Here, the nuts and butter or oil significantly reduce the GI of the rice malt syrup. If you don't have salted butter, add 2 pinches of salt. Don't throw away the baking paper! Sponge it down, fold it neatly and store it to reuse.

COCONUT LEMON CUSTARD TART

SERVES 8 • **PREPARATION TIME** 25 minutes for the pastry, 7–15 minutes for the custard, 2 hours to set • **ACTIVE TIME** 50 minutes ● **GF** ● **VEG** (with agar agar)

You're in for a treat with this tart – the effort is worth it! Check out the photo on page 225.

LEMON CUSTARD FILLING

60–100 ml (2–3½ fl oz) rice malt syrup or maple syrup

2 tablespoons tapioca or arrowroot flour (see note page 210)

2 eggs

2 egg yolks

400 ml (14 fl oz) coconut cream

100 ml (3½ fl oz) filtered water

1 vanilla bean, split lengthways and seeds scraped, or 1 teaspoon vanilla bean powder

2 tablespoons grated lemon zest

juice of 2 lemons

2 level tablespoons powdered gelatine or 1½ tablespoons agar agar

PASTRY

160 g (5¾ oz/1¼ cup) tapioca or arrowroot flour

65 g (2¼ oz/½ cup) buckwheat flour or sorghum flour, plus extra for dusting

35 g (1¼ oz/⅓ cup) almond meal

2 heaped tablespoons coconut flour

140 g (5 oz) salted butter or ghee (frozen for 20 minutes)

2 tablespoons rapadura or panela sugar

1 egg

1 vanilla bean, split lengthways and seeds scraped, or 2 teaspoons vanilla extract

1 teaspoon ground cinnamon

Preheat the oven to 200°C (400°F).

To make the pastry, pulse all the flours in a food processor for about 5 seconds (see note). Add butter and sugar, and pulse for about 5 seconds, until the mixture resembles wet sand. Whisk the egg, vanilla and cinnamon in a bowl. With the motor running, slowly add about two-thirds of this mixture over 3–4 seconds. If it goes to clumps you're done. If not, add a bit more. >>

Lay a sheet of unbleached baking paper (see note page 220) on the benchtop and turn the dough out onto it. Shape into a ball, wrap it in the baking paper and pop in the fridge for 30 minutes to stabilise.

Preheat the oven to 200°C (400°F). Grease a 22 cm (8½ inch) loose-based tart (flan) tin with coconut oil or butter, then dust with buckwheat flour or sorghum flour and shake off any excess. This will help when it comes to dislodging the tart later on.

Plop your pastry blob onto a sheet of baking paper with another sheet on top – both a little longer than the diameter of your tin. Roll the dough out in various directions until it's the diameter of the tin plus 5 cm (2 inches). Peel off the top layer of paper. Turn the bottom paper, with pastry, upside down onto the tin and ease the pastry in, removing the paper and pressing the pastry well into the corner, then trimming off any excess. Pop back in the fridge for another 20 minutes if you have time – pastry is at its absolute best when super chilled. If you have any excess, make a couple of shortbread biscuits (cookies) while you're blind-baking the base. Cook's treat!

Weigh down the paper with baking beads or uncooked rice or dried beans, and blind-bake for 10 minutes with the weights in, then a further 15 minutes without the beads or paper. This will mean your base isn't soggy in the finished product. Once the pastry is a nice medium golden brown, it's ready. Set aside.

Start making the lemon custard when you remove the baking beads from the tart shell. In a medium bowl, whisk the syrup and tapioca flour with the eggs and egg yolks. In a medium saucepan, heat the coconut cream, water, vanilla and lemon zest and juice until just a bubble appears. Pour the hot coconut mixture very, very slowly into the egg mixture, stirring continuously. If you pour too fast, the egg will cook into chunks, and we don't want that! Pour everything straight back into the saucepan and place over medium-low heat, stirring continuously, until the custard thickens. Once thickened, whisk in the gelatine or agar agar, and continue whisking for a few good seconds until incorporated.

If you made your tart shell a while ago and it's cool, cool your custard a little too before filling the shell. Pour your custard into the tart shell. If you have some left, fill a couple of ramekins for a delicious back-up dessert for another day. Let it set in the fridge, only separating base and tin when the tart is fully set; do it carefully and steadily. I never take mine off the base, but just put it on a platter, slice and serve.

Serve nude or with a topping of your choice.

Notes: You can make the pastry in a thermocooker if you have one: mix the flours for 3 seconds on speed 5, then add the butter and sugar, and mix for 3 seconds on speed 6. To make the filling, put in all the ingredients except the gelatine and run for 7 minutes on speed 4, 80°C/175°F, then add the gelatine – 5 seconds on speed 6. You're done.

TOPPING IDEAS

* Cut 4 thin slices of lemon and bake them for 20 minutes in a 180°C (350°F) oven (check at the 15-minute mark). Once they're dried out and sufficiently looking like something from Pinterest, arrange them on the surface of the tart wherever you fancy!

* Drop some blueberries around the tart or to one side as I've done here, with a few edible flowers dotted about for a bit of extra wow factor.

* If you've got loads of spare time, let it set almost completely, then top with a layer of meringue and finish with a blowtorch.

RASPBERRY, MINT AND ROSE JELLIES

SERVES 8 • **COOKING TIME** 15 minutes • **ACTIVE TIME** 20 minutes
● GF ● NF ● EF

For a lighter summer dessert or to serve in tiny glasses as a final touch, these jellies are gorgeous. Free from petroleum-based colours, synthetic sugars and untraceable gelatine, real jelly is therapeutic and delicious. For an added treat, you could top with coconut cream or whipped whole cream.

300 g (10½ oz) fresh raspberries, plus extra to garnish (optional)

375 ml (13 fl oz/1½ cups) cups kombucha or fruit kefir of your choice

60 ml (2 fl oz/¼ cup) maple syrup

90 ml (3 fl oz) boiling filtered water

1 heaped tablespoon powdered gelatine

3 teaspoons rosewater

Place the raspberries, kombucha or kefir and maple syrup in a blender and blend on high for 10 seconds, then pass through a sieve or muslin (cheesecloth) to avoid the chewy raspberry seed vibe (see note).

Heat half the strained liquid in a small saucepan over medium heat until it foams up a little, reserving the other half to add later (this ensures you have some good live bugs still going into your jellies). Pour the water into a small heatproof jug, sprinkle in the gelatine and stir until the gelatine dissolves. Stir the gelatine water into the hot raspberry mixture and remove from the heat. Add the rosewater and the reserved raspberry mixture.

Pour into moulds or a few cute little glasses. Garnish with extra raspberries (if liked). You could also add seasonal edible flowers or mint sprigs, or indeed a mix of all three!

Note: The left-over raspberry pulp is perfect to keep and throw into your next batch of muffins or a tea cake. Freeze it for when that time comes, to avoid waste.

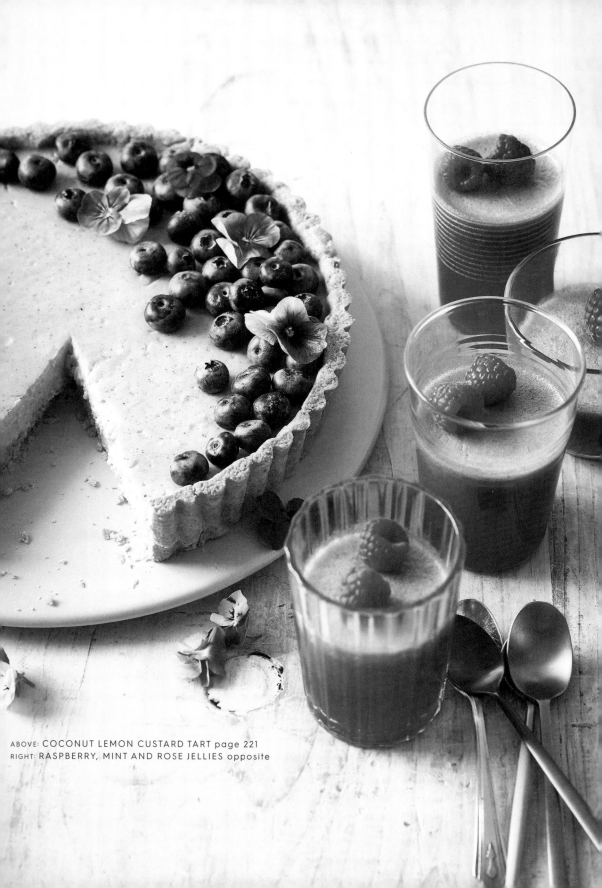

ABOVE: COCONUT LEMON CUSTARD TART page 221
RIGHT: RASPBERRY, MINT AND ROSE JELLIES opposite

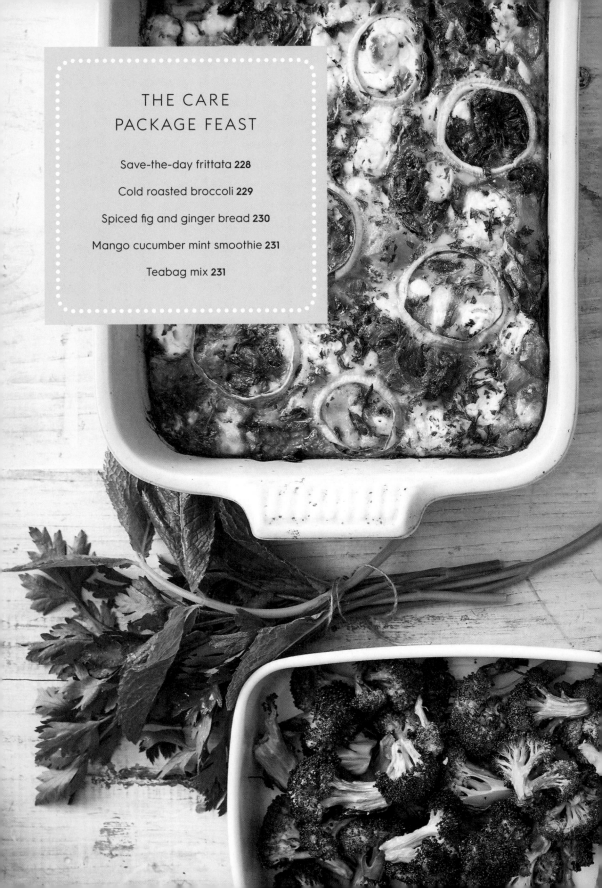

THE CARE PACKAGE FEAST

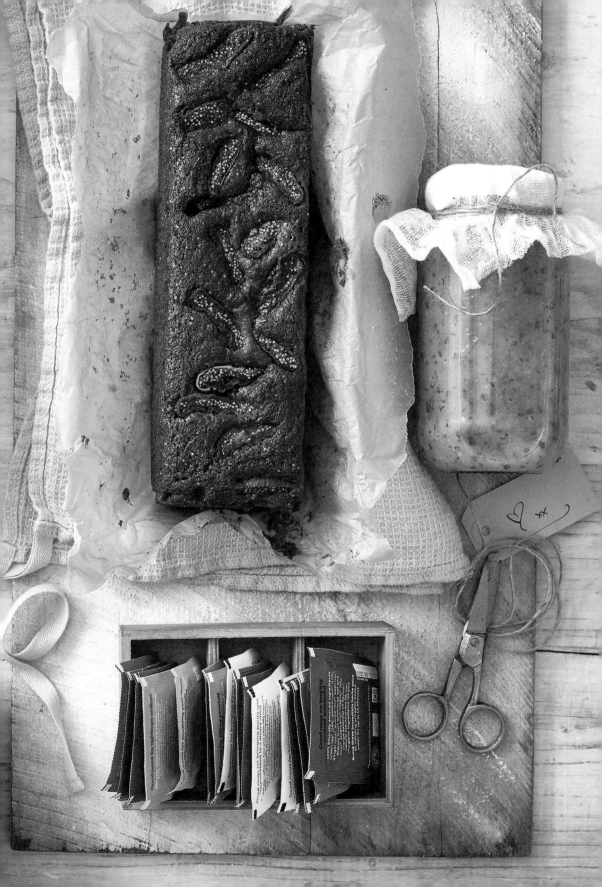

SAVE-THE-DAY FRITTATA

SERVES 10 • **COOKING TIME** 1 hour 40 minutes • **ACTIVE TIME** 20 minutes
● GF ● NF ● VEG

Food gives us such a powerful means to connect and care. Frittata makes the perfect centrepiece for any care package.

140 ml (4¾ fl oz) olive oil

300 g (10½ oz) onions, thinly sliced
   into rounds

700 g (1 lb 9 oz) sweet potato, cut into
   rough 2 cm (¾ inch) cubes

600 g (1 lb 5 oz/about 10) eggs

60 g (2¼ oz/1⅓ cups) rocket (arugula)
   or baby English spinach leaves

120–150 g (4¼–5½ oz) goat's cheese,
   crumbled

½ handful parsley leaves, chopped

1 teaspoon sea salt, or to taste

Preheat the oven to 180°C (350°F).

Heat 2 tablespoons of the olive oil in a large frying pan over medium–high heat and caramelise the onion. Don't overcrowd the pan or you'll end up with soggy onions instead of nicely caramelised ones – if you only have a small frying pan, work in two batches. Turn out into a bowl and set aside.

Spread the sweet potato on a baking tray, drizzle over 60 ml (2 fl oz/ ¼ cup) olive oil and roast for about 1 hour, until soft, checking after 45 minutes. Remove from the oven and set aside to cool. Leave the oven on.

Heat the remaining 2 tablespoons olive oil in a frittata pan. Whisk the eggs well in a large bowl, then pour into the hot pan. Dot the cooled onion and sweet potato all around through the egg, arranging a few onion rings on top. Do the same with the rocket and goat's cheese. Scatter the parsley through the frittata. Don't add salt until the end; salt in eggs while cooking can grey them a little.

Pop in the oven for 30–40 minutes, until there's no wobble in the middle.

Season with salt and serve fresh from the oven or cut into squares whenever food is needed. Because your vegies are packed neatly inside, it's a great stand-alone meal or, for an extra boost, add a salad alongside it.

COLD ROASTED BROCCOLI

MAKES about 100 g (3½ oz) • **COOKING TIME** 25–30 minutes • **ACTIVE TIME** 5 minutes
● GF ● DF ● NF ● EF ● VEG

I love cold roasted veg, and it's perfect for a care package. It's a quick-grab food that's easy on the digestion for a new mum or someone who's unwell, and it can be better than having a lot of raw foods.

1 head broccoli, cut into florets (see note)
60 ml (2 fl oz/¼ cup) olive oil
sea salt, to taste
½ handful mint, or to taste, chopped

Preheat the oven to 200°C (400°F).

Arrange the broccoli florets on a baking tray, taking care not to overcrowd them or they'll be braised and soggy broccoli rather than roasted. If it's crowded, use two trays. Drizzle over the olive oil then mix through with your hands. Sprinkle with salt.

Roast for 25–30 minutes, until the broccoli is crisp and a little golden on some edges.

Scatter over the mint and serve in a bowl or straight from the tray. If putting into a care package, allow to cool then pop into an airtight container.

Note: Set aside the stalks in the freezer for future soups and stews, or roast those too – delicious!

SPICED FIG AND GINGER BREAD

MAKES 1 loaf • **COOKING TIME** 45-55 minutes • **ACTIVE TIME** 10 minutes
● GF ● NF ● VEG

I created this recipe for a lunch with friends, and it's now quite the cult hit.

10 preservative-free dried figs, plus
4–6 extra to garnish

250 ml (9 fl oz/1 cup) boiling filtered
water

2 heaped teaspoons bicarbonate of
soda (baking soda)

100 g (3½ oz) butter or coconut oil,
melted

80–170 ml (2½–5½ fl oz/⅓–⅔ cup) rice
malt syrup or maple syrup, to taste

80 ml (2½ fl oz/⅓ cup) coconut cream

3 eggs

40 g (1½ oz/⅓ cup) coconut flour

90 g (3¼ oz/⅔ cup) buckwheat flour
(try freshly ground), tapioca flour
or arrowroot (see note page 210)

3 teaspoons ground ginger (or more
for ginger-lovers)

1 teaspoon mixed spice (ready-made
or a mix of your own favourites)

Preheat the oven to 180°C (350°F). Grease a loaf (bar) tin about 8 × 25 × 8 cm
(3¼ × 10 × 3¼ inches)/1.6 litres (55½ fl oz) with butter or coconut oil and line
with unbleached baking paper (see note page 220).

Pop the figs in a blender or food processor with the boiling water and
half the bicarbonate of soda. Leave them to soak for 5 minutes. Pour off
170 ml (5½ fl oz/⅔ cup) of the water. Add the butter, syrup, coconut cream
and eggs to the processor, and pulse until smooth. Add the coconut and
buckwheat flours, spices and remaining bicarbonate of soda. Blend for
5–6 seconds on medium.

Pour into the prepared tin. Cut the extra fig into thin strips and arrange
on top. Bake for 45-55 minutes, until a skewer inserted in the centre comes
out clean.

Eat fresh from the oven, or enjoy over the next couple of days toasted and
topped with melting butter or coconut butter, or as little slices in lunchboxes
(nut-free)!

MANGO CUCUMBER MINT SMOOTHIE

SERVES 2–3 • **COOKING TIME** 0 • **ACTIVE TIME** 10 minutes
● GF ● NF ● VEG

This refreshing combination is the perfect pick-me-up for someone who's tired and rundown. Send it in a lovely reusable bottle or sealable carafe.

3 mango cheeks, peeled

1 cucumber

1 handful mint, leaves and thin stalks only (see note)

2 cups (17 fl oz/500 ml) filtered water

juice of 1 lime or ½ lemon (optional)

ice, to serve (optional)

Toss the mango, cucumber and mint in a blender and blitz on high. Add the water and citrus juice (if using), then blend on high for a further for 1 minute, until well mixed and smooth.

Serve on ice or as is. It will last for 2 days in the fridge.

Note: Compost the thicker mint stalks or use them in a soup.

TEABAG MIX

Tea is a gift, materially, health-wise and for the soul. Try these:

* anti-inflammatory teas: tulsi, nettle or lemon balm
* digestive teas: fennel, anise, ginger, mint or nettle
* nursing tea: fenugreek, nettle, marshmallow root, raspberry leaf and fennel.

I can't wait to see us unite online, sharing gifts of love through food to take the load off our friends in need.

CHAPTER FIVE

LOW TOX
MIND

STAYING HAPPY WHILE MAKING LOW TOX CHANGES

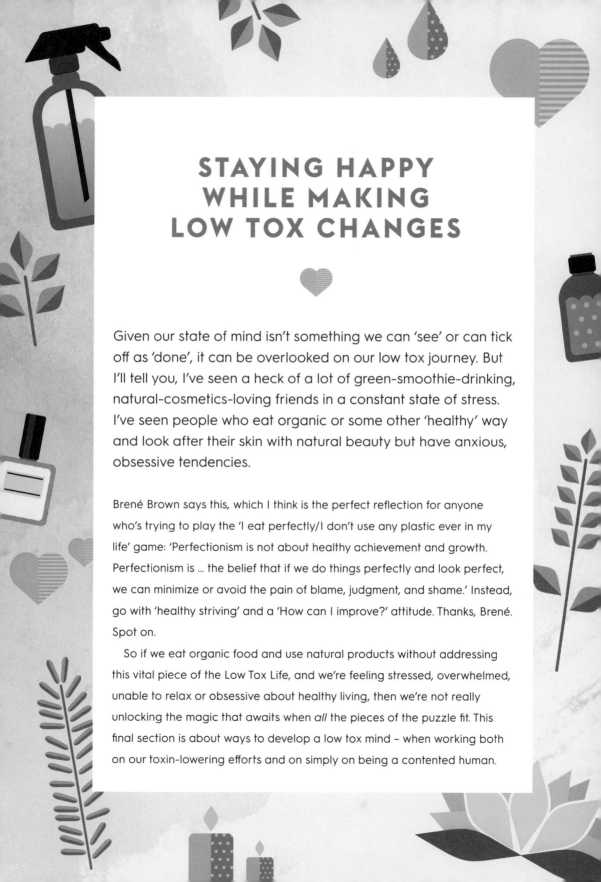

Given our state of mind isn't something we can 'see' or can tick off as 'done', it can be overlooked on our low tox journey. But I'll tell you, I've seen a heck of a lot of green-smoothie-drinking, natural-cosmetics-loving friends in a constant state of stress. I've seen people who eat organic or some other 'healthy' way and look after their skin with natural beauty but have anxious, obsessive tendencies.

Brené Brown says this, which I think is the perfect reflection for anyone who's trying to play the 'I eat perfectly/I don't use any plastic ever in my life' game: 'Perfectionism is not about healthy achievement and growth. Perfectionism is ... the belief that if we do things perfectly and look perfect, we can minimize or avoid the pain of blame, judgment, and shame.' Instead, go with 'healthy striving' and a 'How can I improve?' attitude. Thanks, Brené. Spot on.

So if we eat organic food and use natural products without addressing this vital piece of the Low Tox Life, and we're feeling stressed, overwhelmed, unable to relax or obsessive about healthy living, then we're not really unlocking the magic that awaits when *all* the pieces of the puzzle fit. This final section is about ways to develop a low tox mind – when working both on our toxin-lowering efforts and on simply on being a contented human.

The things our brain has to deal with each day are a huge departure from our natural, wild state. We're so busy processing information these days that there's less thinking and feeling our way through. We're reading ads, catchphrases and headline-only news, and we're forming opinions based on those. We've got 20 tabs open (guilty!) at once. We're doing three different things while we're supposedly playing with or helping our kids. 'Mm-huh, sweetie, Just a second.' Sound familiar? According to a study from the University of California San Diego, we're bombarded with about 34 GB of information per day, or 105,000 words with pictures – enough to burn out the average laptop in a week. Hmmm … burnout. Sounds familiar, and I'm not talking computers, I'm talking *everyone I know at some point*, myself included.

Having a low tox mind is not about denying ourselves the benefits of our connected world and technology – I actually don't know what I'd do raising a child as curious as my son without the support of a search engine. Having a low tox mind is developing certain smarts that become a way and a part of our life – key things we can focus on to find and feel peace every day.

> *Having a low tox mind is not about denying ourselves the benefits of our connected world and technology …*

We can be smarter about what information we choose to consume, and smarter about the tones of voice and words we hear and read, and what we allow into our homes. Next time you scroll through social media feeds, just check in with yourself and ask: 'Is this depleting me or energising me?' Next time you read an article, notice how it affects you. Think about the energy you're bringing into a space. Are you barging in, stressed and grumpy? Or do you take a deep breath before you arrive, and walk in with a smile?

MAKING TIME

We can all be smarter about how we use our abundant 24 hours in each day to our advantage, and to help and enjoy those around us.

OUR TIME FOR US

• • • • • •

We can start to *own* and be comfortable with making quiet time for ourselves. I sent an email newsletter out to our community once, and in it was a beautiful organic, fair-trade coffee giveaway that people could enter. All you had to do was hit reply and share how you best enjoyed your coffee time. You might be thinking, 'Geez, that's a pretty boring competition,' and sure, I could have got more creative, but the responses were fascinating. A few hundred people responded, all women. Except for four entries, every one used the phrases 'steal a bit of' and 'sneak a little' in reference to taking time out just for themselves. Is your mind blown? Think about that for a second. Our time is *ours*, no one else's. We choose to give parts of it to family, friends, causes, work, fitness, TV, emails … ourselves. Yet when it came to making time to chill alone, nearly 100 per cent of my inadvertent small study of 400 test subjects saw time as something that wasn't theirs – something they have to sneak or steal to get and therefore involving guilt or wrongdoing. There's no guilt or wrongdoing in keeping some of your time for yourself. It's *your* time! It's how we have the energy to give so much of it to other people and to our efforts during the day.

There's no guilt or wrongdoing in keeping some of your time for yourself!

It's time for a reframe – time to own our time. It's time to celebrate, connect, find peace, feel grounded and ditch the outdated and harmful thinking that doing so is something to feel guilty about. Here are some ways you might find that time:

* Have a bath and listen to a great podcast or some beautiful music.
* Drink a whole cup of tea before it goes cold.
* Send your partner out with the kids so you can have some peace at home. And do *not* use this precious time to tidy the Lego!
* Read a book.
* Cancel something in your diary that you actually don't want to do and make space for yourself.
* Watch a brilliant movie with some homemade popcorn to accompany it. (*When Harry Met Sally*. Again!)
* Lie in the grass and look up at the trees.
* Play a favourite album and look through old photos (a personal favourite!).
* Meditate (more on that later!).

Do any number of things that refill your cup, but the point is, it's your right and duty to do it, so that you can feel great during the time you give to other people and to must-dos. What if we made recharging ourselves as important a task as recharging our phones? You're not speaking about sneaking time any more. It's yours – and I can't wait to see what excellent investments you make with it.

CONTENTEDNESS

If, as the Dalai Lama says, happiness is not achievable when we're rushed and confused, then no wonder, in this busy modern world, we feel it's around the next corner on hopeful street, rather than something inside us. A calm mind is the only mind that can allow happiness to manifest, he says, so let's find the calm to unlock contentedness.

How can you find contentedness? Rather than trying to 'find' it, decide to *be* it. What can you do? Some journaling, of course! Caveat: I'm not a massive journaler, but at key moments it's exactly what's required.

* Write out a thank-you to your past, citing exact hardships that you often label as having dragged you down, and thank them, because coming through those hardships is what got you here today. My friend Pauline taught me this one, and it's *so* powerful to take the time and say, 'Bye-bye, bitterness.'
* Write a list of the things that make you feel happiness.
* Write a list of your favourite things about yourself – body and character.

Then? Don't waste your precious thoughts and energy on what wasn't great back then, what isn't perfect now, and what would only be better *if*. Just be content. When we're content and grateful, we have everything we need, and therein lies the happiness. When we're happy, we attract a higher vibration – happier people all around us. Contentedness. It's a beautiful thing, as are you.

LOW TOX LIFE

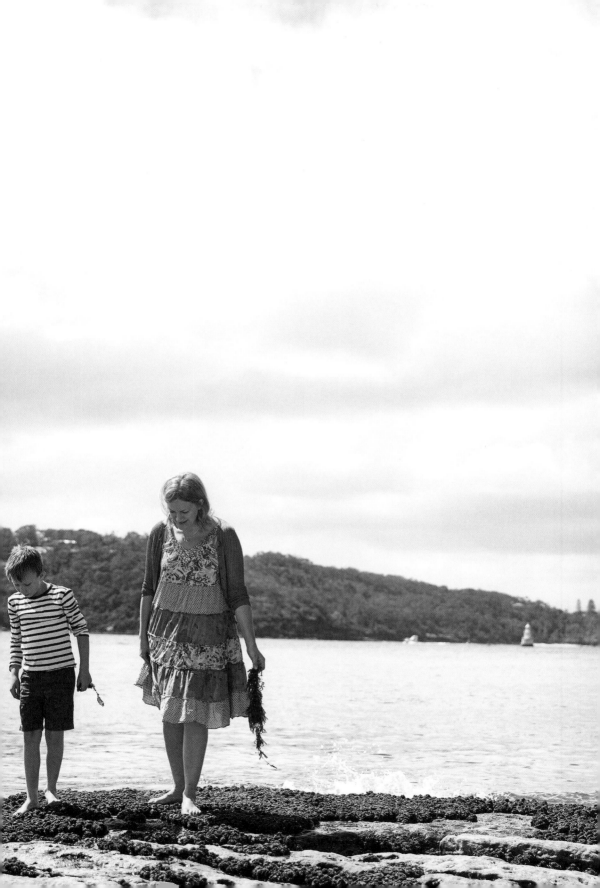

CONNECTEDNESS

When I interviewed Meik Wiking, director of the Happiness Research Institute in Copenhagen and *New York Times* bestselling author of *The Little Book of Hygge*, on the Low Tox Life podcast, we talked a lot about connectedness, joy and cosiness, as you'd imagine. Something he shared really stuck with me, and that was that often when we host people to lunch or dinner we do all the work and we're exhausted, hardly talking to our guests while everyone heralds us as a genius, with praise for the beautiful food or amazing dessert. The meal ends, the guests go home, and we're left with little sense of contentment and connectedness, when being with our friends should be all about those feelings.

He offered the tip the Danes use, which is pot-lucking dinners – where everyone brings something and makes a contribution. There's neither a 'star' nor a workhorse nor someone who didn't lift a finger. Everyone is a part of the creation and the clean-up. Which means that everyone is able to sit, relax, connect and just be instead of running around like a crazy person in the background while the compliments sustain the smile on their flushed-from-cooking face.

   I decided to restart the pot-luck dinners my husband and I used to have pre-child, and I've really felt a much deeper joy in the time I spend with friends as a result. No heroes. No slaves. Everyone in it together and creating a beautiful night. Together.

WHAT CAN WE DO TO FEEL MORE CONNECTED?

. . . . . .

* **Call a friend you haven't spoken to in way too long:** Make a time to catch up. Walks in nature with good friends who never make you feel you need to apologise for who you are? Bliss!

* **Take a meal over to a friend who's going through a tough time:** Spend time being there for them. Feel your heart overflow, even if the tears do too. Listen. Hug. You don't need to fix their problems or have the perfect things to say – just be there. (You might also want to check out my Care Package Feast on page 226.)

* **Put the phone away:** No need to elaborate here – let's just do it more.

* **Hug:** Oxytocin, the luuuurve hormone, can be generated from a hug as little as 20 seconds long. Oxytocin creates optimism and calm, boosts self-esteem, lowers blood pressure and cortisol, creates a sense of trust, and even lowers digestive inflammation. My son and I hug for a good 15 minutes every morning. Luxurious? Yes. Priority for me? Yes. Best start to the day? One hundred per cent.

* **Eat together with the people you love:** Light candles, make sure technology is nowhere to be seen. In an age where fussiness and odd behaviour around food is at crazy levels in kids, eating together not only draws us closer, but allows the kids to see their parents enjoying all the foods parents want their child to eat. Towering over your child saying 'Eat your broccoli!' isn't going to make you or them feel good. Candles lit at a communal table with a big platter in the middle for everyone to serve themselves will provide a backdrop for great eating habits as a family – from both the eating whole foods perspective and the connectedness one. Love a double win!

FEELING EARTHED
AND GROUNDED

There we were at sunrise on a retreat, sitting on the ground in
a small clearing doing some breathing, yoga and meditation.
My wise friend Pauline shared this passage from Vietnamese
monk Thich Nhat Hanh. Once you've read it, get barefoot in
nature. Touch the earth. Feel the godness of it.

"

*In [the Buddhist tradition that I am part of], we do a practice called
'Touching the Earth' every day. It helps us in many ways. You, too,
could be helped by doing this practice. When you feel restless or lack
confidence in yourself, or when you feel angry or unhappy, you can
kneel down and touch the ground deeply with your hand. Touch the
earth as if it were your favorite thing or your best friend.*

*The earth has been there for a long time. She is mother to all of us.
She knows everything. The Buddha asked the earth to be his witness
by touching her with his hand when he had some doubt or fear before
his awakening. The earth appeared to him as a beautiful mother. She
carried flowers and fruit, birds and butterflies, and many different
animals and offered them to the Buddha. The Buddha's doubts and
fears instantly disappeared.*

*Whenever you feel unhappy, come to the earth and ask for her help.
Touch her deeply, the way Buddha did. Suddenly, you too will see
the earth with all her flowers and fruit, trees and birds, animals and
all the living beings that she has produced. All these things she offers
to you.*

"

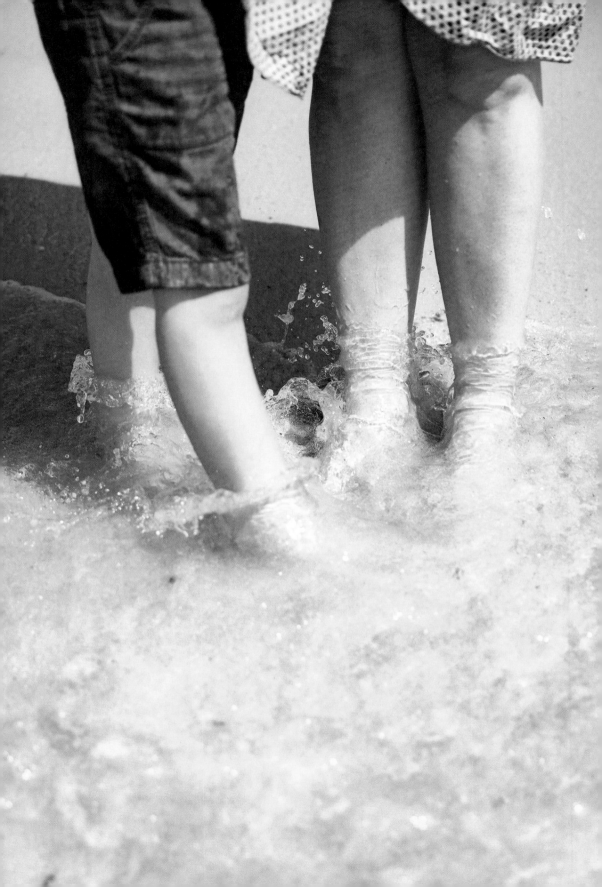

MEDITATION

Are you in the 'I've tried that, it doesn't work' camp? I'm still determined to help you find a way to meditate, as there are so many – you don't have to sit in a corner 'emptying your mind'. (Incidentally, you don't actually have to do this in a sitting meditation. The thoughts will come and you let them float by.)

You don't have to sit in a corner 'emptying your mind'.

MY FOUR FAVOURITE WAYS TO MEDITATE

• • • • • •

1. Standing on the shore of a beach and breathing slow and steady breaths, making music with the sound of the waves lapping onto the shore, over my toes. Nothing beats that for me.

2. Colouring in a mandala as meditation: *Mandala* means 'sacred circle' in Sanskrit. They are often used to assist in meditation, and in sacred sites are used as a transformative, healing tool.

3. Counting backwards from 50 in a quiet place, breathing in for two numbers, out for two, four counts for each breath. To stay with this one, I picture my son at his little desk writing out the numbers as I count backwards and breathe.

4 Doing a yoga nidra meditation: It's a guided meditation you do lying down, moving through and focusing on the different parts of the body. It's a brilliant meditation if you're frazzled or haven't had good sleep, as it's extremely restorative.

OTHER MEDITATION TECHNIQUES TO EXPLORE

* **Vedic meditation:** This is done twice a day, sitting quietly for 20 minutes per session. You focus on a mantra that your teacher gives you, and bring your thoughts back to the mantra each time you stray. There's research to suggest that one session equates to three hours' sleep in terms of bringing your nervous system and brain back into balance.

* **Mindfulness meditation in nature 1:** Slowly put one foot in front of the other, touching your heel to the tip of the toes on your other foot, breathing in for four and out for five, for about 50 steps.

* **Mindfulness meditation in nature 2:** Sit quietly and focus on all that you see and hear around you in nature, one thing at a time. A little bee doing its thing (seriously, how utterly amazing are bees?), the way a leaf is being caught by the breeze, a cloud slowly passing. It's divine.

* **Make a risotto:** Take a leaf out of Nigella Lawson's book and stir, stir, add stock, stir stir, add stock, stir stir, add stock ...

* **Listen to a piece of peaceful music:** Spend time moving through the orchestra, listening to each individual instrument.

* **Do a yin yoga class:** Meditative stretchy and challenging-at-times bliss. You can do these online at home or check out a local studio.

And for goodness sake do not meditate to a guided meditation of a person whose voice you find annoying. So many people give this as their reason for giving up on meditation, but of course you wouldn't like meditation if you didn't find the voice soothing!

REST AND RELAXATION

Make sleep a practice. We must, for it's when we sleep that our brain does its retaining, decluttering and organising, our muscles regenerate and our hormones make their magic. Without sleep we quickly spiral out of control with cravings, lack of creativity, susceptibility to viruses, inability to concentrate, decreased coordination ... and the list goes on.

Your sleep is precious.

Consider implementing a little sleep practice to wind things down each day:

* Cut blue-light exposure a good couple of hours before bed. Get an app for your computer if you're working in the evenings, and use the built-in one on your phone or an app, but do try to work up to less and less tech time in the hour or two before bed.

* Consider sunglasses that block blue light to ensure you're not getting blue light from ambient lights around the house. They're a sexy orange tint. Hey, if you've got a partner and you're both wearing them, everyone's sexy, right?

* Consider switching to candlelight in the evenings. It's so relaxing and calming – exactly the vibes we want before heading to bed.

* Take a book or a magazine to bed with you. I love this because it helps you get out of your own way when it comes to sleep. Channelling my thoughts on a good *New York Times* magazine long form is just about the best way for me to clear my head from my day and get to sleep easily. For you, it might be a good novel.

* Don't exercise too late in the evening, as it can leave your cortisol levels too elevated for you to relax.
* In the bedroom, consider minimal electronics (as we discussed in the bedroom section). The top ones to remove are the digital alarm clock and cordless phone. Switch to an old-school vintage analogue alarm clock, and even try leaving your phone in another part of the house.
* Some people's light sensitivity is so great that they sleep too lightly with ambient light in the room. If that's you, consider a sleep mask and earplugs to ensure you get a good, deep sleep – especially if your partner sleeps with, erm, 'uninhibited, noisy abandon'.
* If you wake in the night, consider having a couple of guided meditations like a yoga nidra loaded onto your phone (if it's in the room) so you can slip the headphones on and do it quietly.
* If you feel you need added support to get to sleep, perhaps a little magnesium could help. Speak to your health practitioner about the best form and dosage. Not all supplements are created equal.
* The more you go, go, go in the day, the harder your body will find it to chill, chill, chill over time. The benefit of taking things down a notch here and there during the day is that you'll find it easier to sleep at night.

If sleep is an issue for you, consider seeing a naturopath or Chinese medicine practitioner to help you find possible root causes and get some herbal or nutrient support. There can be clues as to what is affecting your sleep, based on what time you're waking up and what you experience either when trying to get to sleep (racing mind, wired feeling, loud heart, tinnitus) or when you awake from your sleep (racing heart, sweats, anxiety). Don't let it go unattended! Your sleep is precious, and I'm a big fan of seeing your GP to rule out anything major.

SLOW DOWN

① **Stop eating fast or on the go:** Your digestion cops a beating if you stress and eat at the same time. Same goes for chomping on popcorn during a thriller – it's going to stick there for days! Make eating an intentional practice and please, please, please, teach your kids the same. We don't eat halfway up play equipment, we don't eat running to a meeting. We stop, we eat, we chew at least 25 times per bite to activate the salivary enzymes and start sending messages to our tummies to get gastric juices and bile going. Make the time to stop and chew each bite well.

② **Stop multi-tasking so much:** It's actually a myth that multi-tasking is good for us – it's terrible for you! If you're wondering whether you're experiencing the long-term psychic fallout of too many years of multi-tasking, ask yourself this: 'Do I find it hard to concentrate on just one thing, to be present, to not reach for the phone while at the computer, with ten tabs open, while feeding a child?' Hmmm. *Mini-task:* Leave your phone at home when you go to the shops. Shut all but one window on your computer right now. Sit to read a book and leave your phone off while you do it. Consciously note that you're doing multiple things, and narrow down to a single, pointed focus more and more often, to try it on for size.

③ **Find little pockets of time to breathe in the day:** While washing the dishes or making up a lunchbox, for example. It's funny, but once you approach these 'have-to's as something you know how to do so well that you can do them with your eyes closed, they're an opportunity to relax. It's a brilliant chance to bring a little slow-down into your day and punctuate it with a few good, deep breaths.

4 **Stop telling yourself you're not enough:** You are. *Mini-task*: Every time you give yourself a serving of negative self-talk, force yourself to add double the positive talk. Replace 'I hate my weight' with 'I'm loving that I'm making time for yoga and walks lately'. Where the mind goes, the energy flows!

5 **Remember that we're human beings not human doings:** This favourite quote comes from both Kobe Yamada and Kurt Vonnegut. Every day, take the time to be. Think of the simple act of earthing (page 242) and how good it feels. Let's increase the impact by getting in touch with the mind and taking some slow, deep breaths.

6 **Make a 'stop-doing' list:** My friend and talented yoga teacher Kate Kendall alerted me to this excellent practice. Have a think about your calendar or your 'cram more into the day' tendencies. What can go? A stop-doing list can be a game-changer. Your filter questions are: Is this helpful for me or someone else? Do I enjoy this? Is this adding one thing too many to that day?

7 **Make 'no' a happy word:** Often we say yes only to realise immediately or later that we should have said no. My wise friend Kelly Exeter says, 'Instead, respond by saying, "Let me get back to you," and then you can politely say no the next day.'

PEACEFULLY RADIATING CHANGE

You may have learnt a lot while reading this book. With your new-found knowledge you might want to start speeding through your life and everyone else's around you. You might find you want to shout things from the rooftops. Whoa back! Slow down.

I think anyone who experiences this kind of powerful awakening would be lying if they said they hadn't felt the need to broadcast it all to some degree, but here's the thing: it's essential that your family, partner and close friends don't feel judged or 'wrong', but rather are invited to discover what's really in stuff and discuss how crazy it is that we never knew. Together. You're not against them, you're with them, and you want your children, if you have them, to be healthy and strong, and your partner to feel great and Aunty Cynthia to understand that the plastic throwaway tablecloth, plates and cups for the family Christmas are just not cool.

Happy change is the way you get people on board. If they won't have a bar of it? Just keep doing it for yourself – your life is yours and theirs is theirs. Show off your glowing skin and your energetic vibes, and pretty soon they'll be wondering what you're having and start asking questions! Questions are an invitation for you to speak, and then it feels soft and non-judgy to share a little knowledge.

Happy change is the way you get people on board.

PREACHIN': A SUREFIRE WAY TO LOSE FRIENDS AND PEEVE YOUR FAMILY MEMBERS

• • • • • •

To support your desire for everyone to see instantly what you see, here are five ways to not lose friends or family members while you get busy changing your world:

1 **Consider truthfully why you're doing this:** Share those reasons from the bottom of your heart. If you can connect with your emotional reasons for making these changes, backed by facts, the people around you will be much more likely to see that it's coming from the heart and not just you 'being a pain' or on some 'hippy whacko trip'.

2 **Think before you speak:** You might start to see that it feels like everything and everyone around you is high tox in some way. That's completely normal. It doesn't make you better than them, of course, so it's important to ensure that you create a sense of unity with them, not against them. You might say, for example, 'You know that book I've been reading?' (potential eye-roll or apprehensive 'Yes?') 'Well, it turns out none of these companies are required by law to independently test chemicals for safety before the products are launched. Does that make you want to know what's in it and decide for yourself?' Getting the other person to open up is your best way to work with their enthusiasm and continue to move forward. 'Did you know, for example, that lots of personal-care brands contain hormone-disrupting chemicals? The ones that mimic our own hormones and can make us get hormone-related illnesses? Contributing to infertility? That's really worrying, don't you think?' And a joke always helps: 'It's hard enough to balance our bloody hormones au naturel, without weirdo pretend ones coming in and mucking everything up.'

3 **Watch documentaries together:** You don't want to be secretly learning everything in a corner with 50 tabs open on the internet (I see you!) and then busting out facts passionately and emotionally. You'll sound slightly mad to those around you who were blissfully unaware. I liken it to a break-up – the person who's been thinking for months that this relationship isn't working, planning their future without the other person, planning where they'll move straight after breaking up, does the breaking up. But it's a huge shock for the other person, who is expected to just get on with it after this massive new change. Humans don't like change being inflicted on them, as we all know. And so treat low tox learning as a chance to change together. Let the scientists in the documentaries break the news to you both.

4 **Make it easy for the person resisting:** They may well be afraid that it's all going to be too hard or that it's just not going to be as good. Ask them which 'favourite' products they fear losing, do all the research for them, and make a list of alternatives or buy one for them. Make a care package. Do a 'deodorant performance Olympics', call them the tough Russian judge and get them to score the deodorant replacements you've sourced for them to find the best one to use in the future … Use fun and creativity to foster their buy-in.

5 **Make it delicious:** Taking away a person's favourite biscuits (cookies) with 19 ingredients is still simply taking away a person's biscuits. You're a baddie. Bring them into your delicious new world instead. Bake better, homemade versions. Marvel at the deliciousness of what the real thing tastes like. Discover together that the company was buying cocoa from farms using slave labour, or that to save money on the biscuit's bottom line they're using brown colouring and less chocolate, and that the colouring is derived from petroleum. A few sobering facts coupled with a delicious homemade new treat is far more likely to create sticky change and buy-in than simply saying, 'No more for you!'

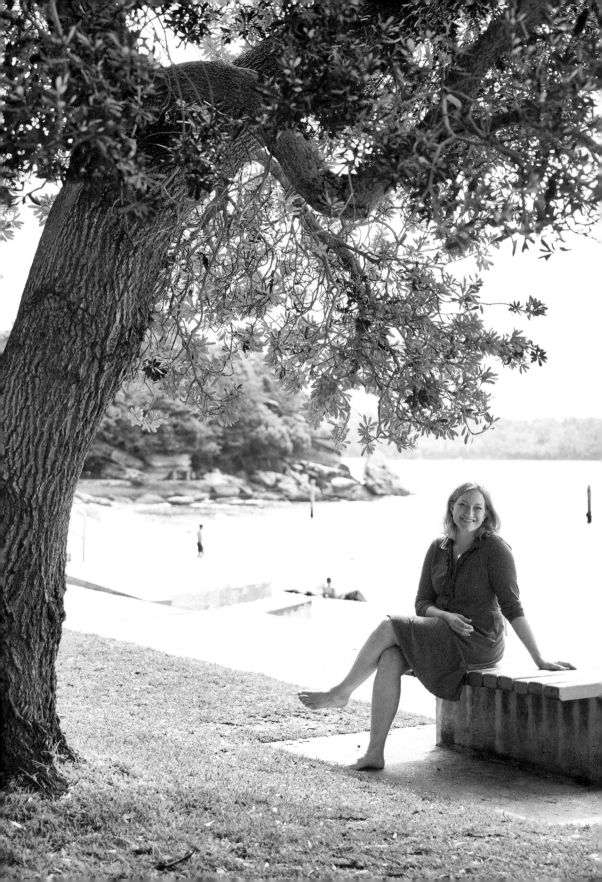

SAMPLE SCRIPTS TO HELP GET YOUR MESSAGE ACROSS

Try adapting these scripts next time an opportunity arises to explain your point of view. Paraphrase them in your own words as you start to make those baby steps towards changing what's in the pantry and fridge, or your personal care and cleaning products. Bringing people along for the ride and planning change together is going to feel so much more exciting than being your household's lone ranger.

SHOPPING WITH A FRIEND

Don't say: 'Ah, that moisturiser you use has parabens. No good.' (Note the accusatory tone.)

Try: 'So I've been researching cosmetics because of this odd rash I was getting sometimes' – there's no need to lie, but sometimes a little white lie makes it less intimidating for you to bring up the natural stuff – 'and I discovered they/the big companies were putting things like X and Y and Z in the stuff we buy. Isn't that crazy? Have you heard about any of this? Anyway, if you want I've done a bit of research and I've found this awesome website XYZ where we can get safe stuff that's really nice-looking/smelling.' (This is inviting and uniting. Feel the difference?)

PARTNER OBJECTION?

Try: 'I've been learning about some of the ways certain ingredients impact the environment, and researching additives that are harmful to us, and it's no good. I'm just going to work over time on substituting better versions of some of the things we've been buying. It means I'll be making more homemade stuff, you'll be pleased to know! I care about all the health problems we hear about and I see all the links between ill health and processed foods, and intensive farming, and some of the chemicals in personal care, and it's worth a shot to avoid certain products where we can, don't you think? Especially if it's just as delicious or easy?'

EMPOWERING THE KIDS

Try: 'Guys, I need your help. I've been learning about some nasty ingredients and want to see if we've got any at home. Will you help me by punching the numbers into this app and seeing if it's a real food ingredient or not? Then we can see if we can learn a new XYZ recipe for anything that comes up with a bad rating. We're not going to lose the treats, we're just going to discover new ones together.' Then make a family Pinterest board and vote for the new treat of the week you're going to make together.

And remember, it's about focusing on yourself as you make changes rather than feeling you must change others. Your radiance and happiness will attract curiosity, and that means you get to play the role of being supportive and offering advice rather than being an 'annoying hippie preacher'.

IT'S NOT GOODBYE, IT'S AU REVOIR

So we're at the end of our time together with this little (okay, it's not that little!) book. I do hope you'll join me in exploring the suggestions at lowtoxlife.com/book-resources if what you've learnt already has whet your appetite for more.

Before I go, though, I'm excited to share a few thoughts on community. Often, when you become aware, you're busting not only to instil the changes in yourself, but to see what you can do to help those around you live a Low Tox Life, for people and the planet.

The more the good stuff grows, the less room there is for the bad, and creating positive change means we remain happy and upbeat in the process, instead of being angry about everything that's wrong. Carve out a beautiful new system, and the old system crumbles. Resisting the system and getting angry about things doesn't seem to be working too well for our collective energy. Bitterness needs to be left at the door. It will be counterproductive to our desire to spread the concept of a Low Tox Life through our communities if we're angry and bitter about everything we see around us.

Carve out a beautiful new system, and the old system crumbles.

Here's how stepping up could look in a few different situations:

✳ **Your parents' group with newborns:** Be the person who knows the best low tox wipes, the good rubber dummy brand, the safe stainless-steel bottles, the most effective and most hassle-free cloth nappies. Establish yourself as the go-to, and you'll get to help all those parents around you.

✳ **Your preschool:** Discuss handwash and sunscreen options with the director of the childcare centre or preschool. Show them the ingredients list of the products they currently use, show the research you've done on the toxic aspects of their ingredients, and suggest alternatives. There's nothing worse than a whinge without a proposed solution.

✳ **Your child's school:** Start working on having the school implement a 'plastic-free lunch' day/nude food day/waste-free Wednesday, as we have, once a week on a permanent basis. Be the parent who offers a list of reusable lunchbox options for the school newsletter (hemp wraps, sandwich pockets, etc.) to help parents find the transition easier. Suggest leftovers for lunch, homemade popcorn in a container rather than packet popcorn (seriously, that stuff is so much more expensive by weight!). Share simple muffin recipes, ideas for crudités and dip, and so on. Again, proposing change without showing the way is not leadership, it's just a statement. We need to help others reskill.

✳ **Your child's high school:** Suggest a sustainability project or that an environmental scientist comes to speak at assembly, with an afternoon workshop to follow. Take3 is a wonderful resource, for example.

✳ **Your child's high school class:** Suggest having them watch a documentary and do research projects on various chemicals and their uses and possible issues. Or get them working on a plan to reduce plastic and paper use in the school. Get kids aware of what's in stuff and its power to affect us – good or bad. You literally change the world, because they grow up doing things differently and knowing exactly why.

✳ **Your sports club or swimming pool:** Campaign for the removal of artificial timed sprays from bathrooms. Suggest alternatives such as diffusing essential oil or simply going without – we survived for decades in public spaces without them. We just don't need them at all. Campaign for low tox washroom and laundry products – there are some great inexpensive options these days. Again, if you have handy the list of dubious ingredients as well as pricing on products to replace them, it's going to make it a lot easier for them to agree.

✳ **Your local cafe:** Encourage them to implement a discount for everyone who brings their own cup. Suggest not serving smoothies in plastic cups when people are 'drinking in'. Ask them to bag up their spent coffee grounds for people to use as body scrubs at home or for their gardens. Discourage the use of straws and make a little sign for the straw pot: 'Every straw ever made still exists. Please only take one if you absolutely need to. Thanks for helping us reduce straw use.'

✳ **Your local restaurant:** There are so many things you can do. Ask them to check with customers before providing straws, and to move to paper straws. All the times a customer says 'No, thanks' are times they'll save money to spend on buying the paper ones instead. Ask them for a doggie bag. If they use plastic tubs for that, let them know there are recycled cardboard options now that are fully compostable. Ask them if they have a compost bin. Raising awareness with a simple question can be the catalyst that the team there needs.

✳ **Your workplace:** Campaign to have auto-timed fragrance fresheners and synthetic scents taken out of work bathrooms. Ask for the company to provide low tox cleaning sprays for the office kitchen, as well as low tox dishwashing liquid, powder and soaps. Make them a list of options. Give them the links to purchase. Make it so easy it would be madness not to. You can also instigate cartridge recycling, low tox commercial cleaning companies, and non-compulsory initiatives like a tai chi morning, weekly yoga class or a 'barefoot lunchtime' initiative. You could give a reusable drink bottle and coffee cup as a start-of-the-year or start-of-employment pack for new staff members.

Here's to starting our little ripples of change, tiny and big, from wherever we are. Who knew that changing our toothpaste and sunscreen could spark us to change the world, eh? So cool. Just begin with you, at your pace, your way, and the rest will all come.

Lastly, I hope, if I did my job right in this book, you've already experienced a few shifts, just reading through. Do you feel a greater sense of place in the world and a drive behind your new-found responsibility for your health and that of our amazing planet earth?

Excitement for discovery rather than fear of the unknown?

Excitement for feeling, deeply, that you're doing something really right – right down to your bones?

Excitement that you're reconnecting to how things are grown and made, how you're feeling and what helps you thrive?

Excitement for nature? We are her and she is us, and respect for nature means we continue to thrive for many generations to come.

So here's to using this book as a springboard to a lifetime of excellent critical thinking, and choices that are better for us and our beautiful planet. Act with the seventh generation in mind, and who knows how quickly we might be able to turn this world around.

Welcome to the new face of activism: peaceful, powerful you!

LOW TOX. HAPPY PEOPLE. HAPPY PLANET.

NOTES

CHAPTER 1: LOW TOX LIFE

22 **more than 140,000 of …:** 'Making our chemical future green and clean', UN Environment, drustage. unep.org/environmentalgovernance/making-our-chemical-future-green-and-clean

23 **According to the Ocean Cleanup research team …:** Ocean Cleanup, www.theoceancleanup.com

Today, the US Centers …: 'Autism spectrum disorder', CDC, US, www.cdc.gov/ncbddd/autism/data.html

In November 2015, …: B. Zablotsky et al., 'Estimated prevalence of autism and other developmental disabilities following questionnaire changes in the 2014 National Health Interview Survey', *National Health Statistics Reports*, 13 November 2015, no. 87, www.cdc.gov/nchs/data/nhsr/nhsr087.pdf

Every day, 8 trillion …: C.M. Rochman et al., 'Scientific evidence supports a ban on microbeads', *Environmental Science and Technology*, 2015, vol. 49, pp. 10759-61.

24 **One in five of us …:** ABS, 'Summary of findings: prevalence of mental disorders', 4326.0 – National Survey of Mental Health and Wellbeing: Summary of Results, 2007; NIH, US, 'Any mental illness (AMI) among U.S. adults', www.nimh.nih.gov/health/statistics/prevalence/any-mental-illness-ami-among-us-adults.shtml; NHS, UK, 'Adult psychiatric morbidity in England', digital.nhs.uk/catalogue/PUB02931

Reports from several countries state …: Ming-Ho Yu et al., *Environmental Toxicology: Biological and Health Effects of Pollutants*, 3rd edn, CRC Press, Boca Raton, Florida, p. 69.

as many as one in six …: M.E. Thoma, et al., 'Prevalence of infertility in the United States as estimated by the current duration approach and a traditional constructed approach', *Fertility and Sterility*, 2013, vol. 99, no. 5, pp. 1324-31.

This is an increase from the 1995 figure …: ABS, 'Overweight and obesity', 4364.0.55.001 – National Health Survey: First Results, 2014-15.

The current incarnations of the commonly used pesticides …: UN General Assembly, 'Report of the Special Rapporteur on the right to food', Human Rights Council, 34th session, 27 February – 24 March 2017, documents-dds-ny.un.org/doc/UNDOC/GEN/G17/017/85/pdf/G1701785.pdf?OpenElement

In the past decade, Australia, …: S. Berterame, 'Use of and barriers to access to opioid analgesics: a worldwide, regional, and national study', *Lancet*, 2016, vol. 387, no. 10028, pp. 1644-56.

Currently, nine in ten deaths in Australia …: *Australia's Health 2014*, AIHW, Canberra, 2014, www.aihw.gov.au/getmedia/8f7bd3d6-9e69-40c1-b7a8-40dca09a13bf/4_2-chronic-disease.pdf.aspx

According to the US Environmental Protection Agency …: Zhai Yun Tan, 'What happens when fashion becomes fast, disposable and cheap?', NPR, 10 April 2016, www.npr.org/2016/04/08/473513620/what-happens-when-fashion-becomes-fast-disposable-and-cheap

On average we each throw out …: Council for Textile Recycling, www.weardonaterecycle.org

CHAPTER 2: LOW TOX BODY

40 **And they can block or interfere with …:** 'Endocrine disruptors', NIEHS, NIH, US, www.niehs.nih.gov/health/topics/agents/endocrine/index.cfm

Endocrine disruptors affect multiple systems …: 'Children's environmental health: endocrine disrupting chemicals (EDCs)', WHO, www.who.int/ceh/risks/cehemerging2/en

More recently, they've …: F. Grün & B. Blumberg, 'Environmental obesogens: organotins and endocrine disruption via nuclear receptor signaling', *Endocrinology*, 2006, vol. 147, no. 6 suppl., pp. S50-55.

41 **In 2009 the Endocrine Society …:** E. Diamanti-Kandarakis et al., 'Endocrine disrupting chemicals: An Endocrine Society scientific statement', Endocrine Society, 2009, www.endocrine.org/-/media/endosociety/files/publications/scientific-statements/edc_scientific_statement.pdf

The good news about phthalates …: W.J. Crinnion, 'Toxic effects of the easily avoidable phthalates and parabens', *Alternative Medicine Review*, 2010, vol. 15, no. 3, pp. 190-96.

The available research studies show ...: J.D. Meeker, 'Exposure to environmental endocrine disruptors and child development', *Archives of Pediatric and Adolescent Medicine*, 2012, vol. 166, no. 6, pp. E1–E7.

42   **They've been detected in human breast cancer tissues** ...: P.D. Darbre et al., 'Concentrations of parabens in human breast tumours', *Journal of Applied Toxicology*, 2004, vol. 24. no. 1, pp. 5–13.

Parabens may also interfere ...: S. Oishi, 'Effects of propyl paraben on the male reproductive system', *Food and Chemical Toxicology*, 2002, vol. 40, no. 12, pp. 1807–13.

Some studies say this is safe ...: Scientific Committee on Consumer Safety (SCCS), 'Opinion of the Scientific Committee on Consumer Safety (SCCS) – final version of the opinion on phenoxyethanol in cosmetic products', *Regulatory Toxicology and Pharmacology*, 2016, vol. 82, no. 156.

The Dow Chemical safety data sheet ...: Dow, 'Ethylene glycol phenyl ether', rev. 8 November 2016, msdssearch.dow.com/PublishedLiteratureDOWCOM/dh_0977/0901b80380977062.pdf?filepath=productsafety/pdfs/noreg/233-00323.pdf&fromPage=GetDoc

Resourcinol: A hormone disruptor found in ...: BKH Consulting Engineers & TNO Nutrition and Food Research, 'Annex 13: List of 146 substances with endocrine disruption classifications prepared in the Expert meeting', in 'Towards the establishment of a priority list of substances for further evaluation of their role in endocrine disruption', European Commission Directorate-General for Environment, ec.europa.eu/environment/archives/docum/pdf/bkh_annex_13.pdf

43   **Benzophinone: A possible hormone disruptor** ...: S. Kim et al., 'Effects of benzophenone-3 exposure on endocrine disruption and reproduction of Japanese medaka (*Oryzias latipes*) – a two generation exposure study', *Aquatoxicology*, 2014, vol. 155, pp. 244–52.

Triphenyl phosphate: An endocrine disruptor used mostly ...: J. Congleton, 'Nailed: endocrine disruptor in nail polishes gets into women's bodies', EWG, 19 October 2015, www.ewg.org/research/nailed

Research shows that constant exposure ...: E. Mendelsohn et al. (including J. Congleton), 'Nail polish as a source of exposure to triphenyl phosphate', *Environment International*, 2016, vol. 86, pp. 45–51.

Skin irritants both, and the latter ...: C.A.M. Bondi et al., 'Human and environmental toxicity of sodium lauryl sulfate (SLS): evidence for safe use in household cleaning products', *Environmental Health Insights*, 2015, vol. 9, pp. 27–32.

Damaging to the thyroid gland ...: R.J. Witorsch, 'Critical analysis of endocrine disruptive activity of triclosan and its relevance to human exposure through the use of personal care products', *Critical Reviews in Toxicology*, 2014, vol. 44, no. 6, pp. 535–55.

These are a common cause of eczema ...: A. Wibbertmann et al., *Benzoic Acid and Sodium Benzoate*, WHO, Geneva, 2000, www.who.int/ipcs/publications/cicad/cicad26_rev_1.pdf

a known eye irritant ...: G.H.Y. Lin & M. Hemming, 'Ocular and dermal irritation studies of some quaternary ammonium compounds', *Food Chemical Toxicology*, 1996, vol. 34, no. 2, pp. 177–82.

44   **It has caused a marked rise in** ...: J.L. Cahill et al., 'Methylisothiazolinone in baby wipes: a rising star among causes of contact dermatitis', *Medical Journal of Australia*, 2014, vol. 200, no. 4, p. 208.

These similar chemicals ...: B. Nair, 'Final report on the safety assessment of benzyl alcohol, benzoic acid, and sodium benzoate', *International Journal of Toxicology*, 2010, vol. 20, supplement no. 3, pp. 23–50.

EWG has found it to ...: '1,4-dioxane', EWG, www.ewg.org/skindeep/ingredient/726331/1,4-DIOXANE

47   **According to some sources, the three** ...: J. Sarkissian, 'Mouth breathing', DDS Sarkissian Biological and Homeopathic Dentistry, www.sarkissiandds.com/articles/1009.html

48   **shown to support skin tone** ...: Hsin-Yi Peng et al., 'Effect of *Vetiveria zizanioides* essential oil on melanogenesis in melanoma cells: downregulation of tyrosinase expression and suppression of oxidative stress', *Scientific World Journal*, 2014, vol. 2014, article no. 213013.

56   **This mineral has inconclusive yet strong** ...: J.E. Muscat et al., 'Perineal talc use and ovarian cancer: a critical review', *European Journal of Cancer Prevention*, 2008, vol. 17, no. 2, pp. 139–46.

57   **Cadmium is a carcinogen that has been found** ...: J.G. Ionescu et al., 'Increased levels of transition metals in breast cancer tissue', *Neuroendocrinology Letters*, 2006, vol. 27, supplement no. 1, pp. 36–39.

these can accumulate …: S. De Coster & N. van Larebeke, 'Endocrine-disrupting chemicals: associated disorders and mechanisms of action', *Journal of Environmental and Public Health*, vol. 2012, no. 713696.

Chronic exposure is linked to anaemia …: J.M. Donald et al., 'Reproductive and developmental toxicity of toluene: a review', *Environmental Health Perspectives*, 1991, vol. 94, pp. 237–44.

can possibly accumulate in our tissues …: N. Concin et al., 'Evidence for Cosmetics as a Source of Mineral Oil Contamination in Women', *Journal of Women's Health*, 2011, vol. 20, no. 11, pp. 1713–19.

tamper with our oestrogen levels: P. Tarnow et al., 'Estrogenic activity of mineral oil aromatic hydrocarbons used in printing inks', *PLOS ONE*, 2016, vol. 11, no. 1, article no. e0147239.

58   **Butylated hydroxyanisole … are thought to be …**: A. Pop et al., 'Endocrine disrupting effects of butylated hydroxyanisole (BHA – E320)', *Clujul Medical*, 2013, vol. 86, no. 1, pp. 16–20.

They are suspected endocrine disruptors …: 'Cyclotetrasiloxane', EWG, www.ewg.org/skindeep/ingredient/701743/CYCLOTETRASILOXANE/ - .WhOkChJ96b8

And they're harmful to fish …: 'The dirty dozen: siloxanes', David Suzuki Foundation, davidsuzuki.org/issues/health/science/toxics/chemicals-in-your-cosmetics---siloxanes

Often found in SPF face powders …: European Commission Scientific Committee on Emerging and Newly Identified Health Risks (SCENIHR), 'Nanotechnologies', 2006, ec.europa.eu/health/scientific_committees/opinions_layman/en/nanotechnologies/l-2/6-health-effects-nanoparticles.htm; M. Cimitile, 'Nanoparticles in sunscreen damage microbes', *Scientific American*, 24 March 2009, www.scientificamerican.com/article/nanoparticles-in-sunscreen

62   **All of these oils are brilliant …**: B. Ali et al., 'Essential oils used in aromatherapy: a systemic review', *Asian Pacific Journal of Tropical Biomedicine*, 2015, vol. 5, no. 8, pp. 601–11.

64   **benzalkonium chloride: This is …**: 'Benzalkonium chloride compounds', Toxnet, NIH, US National Library of Medicine, 13 May 2010, toxnet.nlm.nih.gov/cgi-bin/sis/search/a?dbs+hsdb:@term+@DOCNO+234

triclosan: We already …: S.E. Anderson & B.J. Meade, 'Potential health effects associated with dermal exposure to occupational chemicals', *Environmental Health Insights*, 2014, vol. 8, supplement no. 1, pp. 51–62; 'Not effective and not safe: the FDA must regulate dangerous antimicrobials in everyday products', Natural Resources Defense Council, www.nrdc.org/sites/default/files/antimicrobials.pdf

66   **OMC easily penetrates the upper layer …**: N. Duale et al., 'Octyl methoxycinnamate modulates gene expression and prevents cyclobutane pyrimidine dimer formation but not oxidative DNA damage in UV-exposed human cell lines', *Toxicological Sciences*, 2010, vol. 114, no. 2, pp. 272–84.

Male rats born to mothers exposed …: M. Schlumpf et al., 'Developmental toxicity of UV filters and environmental exposure: a review', *International Journal of Andrology*, 2008, vol. 31. no. 2, pp. 144–51.

Human trials found that both OMC and 4-MBC …: J.A. Ruszkiewicz et al., 'Neurotoxic effect of active ingredients in sunscreen products: a contemporary review', *Toxicology Reports*, 2017, vol. 4, pp. 245–59.

When exposed to sunlight, this generates …: 'Padimate O', EWG, www.ewg.org/skindeep/ingredient/704392/PADIMATE_O/ - .WhOxDxJ96b8

67   **we're meant to sweat …**: S.J. Genuis, 'Blood, urine, and sweat (BUS) study: monitoring and elimination of bioaccumulated toxic elements', *Archives of Environmental Contamination and Toxicology*, 2011, vol. 61, no. 2, pp. 344–57.

68   **They could both be toxic if absorbed …**: 'Diethanolamine', Toxnet, 15 May 2014, toxnet.nlm.nih.gov/cgi-bin/sis/search/a?dbs+hsdb:@term+@DOCNO+924; 'Triethanolamine', Toxnet, 22 September 2016, toxnet.nlm.nih.gov/cgi-bin/sis/search/a?dbs+hsdb:@term+@DOCNO+893

They are already restricted …: 'Ethanolamine compounds', Campaign for Safe Cosmetics, www.safecosmetics.org/get-the-facts/chemicals-of-concern/ethanolamine-compounds

Some of these synthetic colours …: S. Kobylewski & M.F. Jacobson, 'Toxicology of food dyes', *International Journal of Occupational and Environmental Health*, 2012, vol. 18, no. 3, pp. 220–46.

they also often cause …: 'Food dye can cause severe allergic reactions', 25 January 2007, University of Michigan, ns.umich.edu/new/releases/1760-food-dye-can-cause-severe-allergic-reactions

69 **We're thought, on average, to use 12,000 …:** F. Edraki, 'Tampons, pads, menstrual cups, period underwear: what's best for the environment?', updated 4 November 2017, ABC News, www.abc.net.au/news/2017-10-27/which-period-product-is-best-for-the-environment/9090658

Because of their cotton content …: A. Donsky, 'Is there pesticide residue on your tampons? Our independent testing gets specific', Naturally Savvy, naturallysavvy.com/care/is-there-pesticide-residue-on-your-tampons-our-independent-testing-gets-specific; *Robin Danielson Act 2008*, H.R.5181, 110th US Congress, www.congress.gov/bill/110th-congress/house-bill/5181/text

78 **This has been called …:** R.T. Zoeller et al., 'Endocrine-disrupting chemicals and public health protection: a statement of principles from the Endocrine Society', *Endocrinology*, 2012, vol. 153, no. 9, pp. 4097–110.

82 **is suspected of reproductive …:** M.D. Reuber, 'Carcinogenicity of saccharin', *Environmental Health Perspectives*, 1978, vol. 25, pp. 173–200.

84 **Given that Americans use around 4.3 million kilometres …:** K.S. Kruszelnicki, 'Dental Floss 1', 30 March 2001, ABC Science, www.abc.net.au/science/articles/2001/03/30/268342.htm

91 **There's a lot of research on coriander …:** M. Aga et al., 'Preventive effect of *Coriandrum sativum* (Chinese parsley) on localized lead deposition in ICR mice', *Journal of Ethnopharmacology*, 2001, vol. 77, nos 2–3, pp. 203–208.

CHAPTER 3: LOW TOX HOME

98 **They are endocrine disruptive to …:** R. Morgenstern et al., 'Phthalates and thyroid function in preschool age children: sex specific associations', *Environment International*, 2017, vol. 106, pp. 11–18; J.D. Meeker et al., 'Di(2-ethylhexyl) phthalate metabolites may alter thyroid hormone levels in men', *Environmental Health Perspectives*, 2007, vol. 115, no. 7, pp. 1029–34; S. Sedha et al., 'Role of oxidative stress in male reproductive dysfunctions with reference to phthalate compounds', *Urology Journal*, 2015, vol. 12, no. 5, pp. 2304–16; A. Karwacka et al., 'Exposure to modern, widespread environmental endocrine disrupting chemicals and their effect on the reproductive potential of women: an overview of current epidemiological evidence', *Human Fertility*, 2017, vol. 31, pp. 1–24.

Triclosan can disrupt …: E.M. Rees Clayton et al., 'The impact of bisphenol A and triclosan on immune parameters in the U.S. population', *Environmental Health Perspectives*, 2011, vol. 119, pp. 390–96.

Studies have called for urgent further research …: N. Tatarazako et al., 'Effects of triclosan on various aquatic organisms', *Environmental Sciences*, 2004, vol. 11, no. 2, pp. 133–40.

In addition to causing lung irritation when inhaled …: '2-butoxyehtanol', 12 August 1996, hazard.com/msds/mf/baker/baker/files/b6100.htm

Dr Rebecca Sutton …: J. Sholl, '8 hidden toxins: what's lurking in your cleaning products?', Experience Life, October 2011, experiencelife.com/article/8-hidden-toxins-whats-lurking-in-your-cleaning-products

'Although the EPA sets a standard …': 'Glycol ethers', EPA safety data sheet, www.epa.gov/sites/production/files/2016-09/documents/glycol-ethers.pdf

99 **'Ammonia is a powerful irritant …':** V.R. Thrane et al., 'Ammonia triggers neuronal disinhibition and seizures by impairing astrocyte potassium buffering', *Nature Medicine*, 2013, vol. 19, pp. 1643–48.

These can be acute …: Jiang-Hua Li, 'Health effects from swimming training in chlorinated pools and the corresponding metabolic stress pathways', *PLOS ONE*, 2015, vol. 10, no. 3, article no. e0119241.

100 **A real problem with sodium laureth …:** C.A.M. Bondi, 'Human and environmental toxicity of sodium lauryl sulfate (SLS): evidence for safe use in household cleaning products', *Environmental Health Insights*, 2015, vol. 9, pp. 27–32.

Napthas, depending on regularity …: 'Hazardous substance fact sheet: naphtha', New Jersey Department of Health and Senior Services, nj.gov/health/eoh/rtkweb/documents/fs/0518.pdf

They can also be contaminated …: 'Naphtha', www.collectioncare.org/MSDS/naphthamsds.pdf

101 **Safety data sheets …:** 'Safety data sheet … optical brightening agent TF-351', Orica, 12 August 2009, msds.orica.com/pdf/shess-en-cds-010-000000018959.pdf

and they can cause ...: allergic reactions: J.L. Marks, 'Quantifying the transfer of optical brighteners from fabric to skin', MSc thesis, University of Washington, 2015

These operate similarly to triclosan ...: A. Bello et al., 'Characterization of occupational exposures to cleaning products used for common cleaning tasks-a pilot study of hospital cleaners', *Environmental Health*, 2009, vol. 8, article no. 11.

benzyl acetate (possibly ...): D.S. Longnecker et al., 'Evaluation of promotion of pancreatic carcinogenesis in rats by benzyl acetate', *Food and Chemical Toxicology*, 1990, vol. 28, no. 10, pp. 665–68.

benzyl alcohol (can irritate ...): 'Benzyl alcohol: sc-326216', chemical safety data sheet, 20 August 2009, at Santa Cruz Biotechnology, datasheets.scbt.com/sc-326216.pdf

chloroform (a neurotoxin ...): 'Chloroform', EPA safety data sheet, www.epa.gov/sites/production/files/2016-09/documents/chloroform.pdf

105   **Did you know that ...**: 'Please don't use bleach', Mycologia, www.mycologia.com.au/don't-use-bleach

115   **it's listed as a carcinogen**: 'Tetrachloroethylene (Perchloroethylene)', EPA safety data sheet, www.epa.gov/sites/production/files/2016-09/documents/tetrachloroethylene.pdf

117   **Stainless-steel pans containing nickel ...**: 'Nickel allergy', Healthline, www.healthline.com/health/allergies/nickel - symptoms2

      Copper pans (which can raise ...): 'Council of Europe's policy statements concerning materials and articles intended to come into contact with foodstuffs', 13 February 2002, at Mast: Icelandic Food and Veterinary Authority, www.mast.is/Uploads/document/guidelines_metals_alloys_used_as_food_contact_materials.pdf

125   **research shows that water ...**: 'Bottled waters contaminated with antimony from PET', press release, 24 January 2006, University of Heidelberg, www.uni-heidelberg.de/press/news/news06/2601antime.html

      This isn't counting the fuel ...: Pacific Institute, 'Fact sheet: bottled water and energy – getting to 17 million barrels', December 2007, no longer online.

      That's more than $1 billion ...: C. Fishman, 'Message in a bottle', Fast Company magazine, 1 July 2007, p. 110, www.fastcompany.com/59971/message-bottle

      PET plastic bottles can ...: W. Shotyk et al., 'Contamination of Canadian and European bottled waters with antimony from PET containers', *Journal of Environmental Monitoring*, 2006, vol. 8, no. 2, pp. 288–92.

126   **In 2002 alone, 5 trillion plastic bags ...**: 'Plastic bags used per year', The World Counts, www.theworldcounts.com/counters/waste_pollution_facts/plastic_bags_used_per_year

      alternatives like BPF ...: C.Z. Yang et al., 'Most plastic products release estrogenic chemicals: a potential health problem that can be solved', *Environmental Health Perspectives*, 2011, vol. 119, pp. 989–96.

      There's more and more evidence ...: 'Exposure to BPA substitute, BPS, multiplies breast cancer cells', Science News, Science Daily, 3 April 2017, www.sciencedaily.com/releases/2017/04/170403140605.htm

127   **Roughly 50 per cent ...**: 'The facts are overwhelming', Plastic Oceans, www.plasticoceans.org/the-facts

      The amount of plastic ...: N. D'Alessandro, '22 facts about plastic pollution', 7 April 2014, EcoWatch, www.ecowatch.com/22-facts-about-plastic-pollution-and-10-things-we-can-do-about-it-1881885971.html

      Throughout the world, around 1 million ...: 'Marine debris', Australian Marine Conservation Society, www.marineconservation.org.au/pages/marine-debris.html

136   **In Australia, 3.28 million tonnes ...**: 'Environmental impact: food waste in Australia', Foodbank, www.foodbanknsw.org.au/about-us/environmental-impact

      In the United Kingdom ...: A. Cowburn, 'UK households wasted 7.3 million tonnes of food in 2015, new figures reveal', 10 January 2017, *Independent*, www.independent.co.uk/news/uk/part-mp-a7517931.html

      In the United States ...: S. Goldenberg, 'Half of all US food produce is thrown away, new research suggests', 13 July 2016, *Guardian*, theguardian.com/environment/2016/jul/13/us-food-waste-ugly-fruit-vegetables-perfect?CMP=share_btn_tw

145   **Although not technically a heavy metal ...**: R.A. Yokel, 'The toxicology of aluminum in the brain: a review', *Neurotoxicology*, 2000, vol. 21, no. 5, pp. 813–28; Stephen C. Bondy, 'The neurotoxicity of environmental aluminum is still an issue', *Neurotoxicology*, 2010, vol. 31, no. 5, pp. 575–81.

148 **particularly for the 24 ...**: 'HLA DR', SurvivingMold, www.survivingmold.com/diagnosis/lab-tests
The potential symptom list is long ...: 'Common mold sickness misdiagnoses', SurvivingMold, www.survivingmold.com/mold-symptoms/common-mold-sickness-misdiagnoses-is-this-really-my-illness-1

150 **including one by the World Health Organization ...**: 'Electromagnetic fields and public health: mobile phones', fact sheet no. 193, reviewed October 2014, WHO, www.who.int/mediacentre/factsheets/fs193/en

158 **Consider that Australians buy ...**: J. Milburn, 'Aussies send 85% of textiles to landfill', Textile Beat, 18 August 2016, textilebeat.com/aussies-send-85-of-textiles-to-landfill
Or that Americans collectively throw away ...: G. Frazee, 'How to stop 13 million tons of clothing from getting trashed every year', PBS News Hour, 7 June 2016, www.pbs.org/newshour/nation/how-to-stop-13-million-tons-of-clothing-from-getting-trashed-every-year
Between 1980 and 2014 ...: E. Cline, 'Where does discarded clothing go?', The Atlantic, 18 July 2014, www.theatlantic.com/business/archive/2014/07/where-does-discarded-clothing-go/374613
In 2014, 55.2 ...: A. Carmichael, 'Man-made fibers continue to grow', Textile World, January/February 2015, www.textileworld.com/textile-world/fiber-world/2015/02/man-made-fibers-continue-to-grow
They now show up in everything ...: S. Howard, 'Environmental awareness', 5 January 2017, School of Public Health, University of Minnesota, www.sph.umn.edu/news/environmental-awareness

160 **When it comes to shoes, a UK study ...**: G. Allen, 'Women own 21 pairs of shoes on average', Mirror (London), 8 October 2014, www.mirror.co.uk/news/uk-news/women-21-pairs-shoes-average-4400118

CHAPTER 4: LOW TOX FOOD

172 **Studies have demonstrated that colours ...**: L.E. Arnold et al., 'Artificial food colors and attention-deficit/ hyperactivity symptoms: conclusions to dye for', Neurotherapeutics, 2012, vol. 9, no. 3, pp. 599–609.

173 **residues from said herbicide have been shown ...**: R. Mesnage et al., 'Multiomics reveal non-alcoholic fatty liver disease in rats following chronic exposure to an ultra-low dose of Roundup herbicide', Scientific Reports, vol. 7, article no. 39328,.
It's thought that up to 60 per cent ...: J. Higdon et al., 'Folate', Micronutrient Information Center, Linus Pauling Institute, Oregon State University, 2000 with updates, lpi.oregonstate.edu/mic/vitamins/folate
These are known to affect sensitive people ...: See, for example, H. Vally et al., 'Clinical effects of sulphite additives', Clinical and Experimental Allergy, 2009, vol. 39, no. 1, pp. 1643–51.
These have been shown to suppress female ...: M. Mondal et al., 'Monosodium glutamate suppresses the female reproductive function by impairing the functions of ovary and uterus in rat', Environmental Toxicology, 2017, online pre-publication, doi: 10.1002/tox.22508.
Studies show that consumers of artificial sweeteners ...: M.R. Ardalan et al., 'Nephrotoxic effect of aspartame as an artificial sweetener', Iranian Journal of Kidney Diseases, 2017, vol. 11, no. 5.

174 **long-term plastic food storage ...**: M. Wagner & J. Oehlmann, 'Endocrine disruptors in bottled mineral water: total estrogenic burden and migration from plastic bottles', Environmental Science and Pollution Research, 2009, vol. 16, no. 3, pp. 278–86.

CHAPTER 5: LOW TOX MIND

234 **'Perfectionism is not about healthy ...'**: B. Brown, Daring Greatly, Penguin, London, 2015, pp. 130–31.

235 **According to a study from the University of California ...**: D. Ramsey, 'UC San Diego experts calculate how much information Americans consume: computer games and TV account for bulk of information consumed in 2008', 9 December 2009, UC San Diego News Center, ucsdnews.ucsd.edu/archive/newsrel/general/12-09Information.asp

241 **Oxytocin creates optimism ...**: For links to relevant scientific articles, see Alejandra 'Alex' Ruani, 'Hugs, the ultimate vaccine', Health Sciensces Academy, thehealthsciencesacademy.org/health-tips/hugs

242 **'In [the Buddhist tradition ...'**: Thich Nhat Hanh, 'Touching the Earth', A Pebble for Your Pocket: Mindful Stories for Children and Grown-ups, Plum Blossom Books, Berkeley, California, 2001, pp. 93–94.

ACKNOWLEDGEMENTS

It takes a team of people to bring a baby into the world - and it turns out a book is no different!

Thanks to Ollie - you were there for cuddles and workshopping stuck-ness when I needed it, and whisked our beautiful son off on a camping trip when I needed time to write. I appreciate and love you so much, *chéri*.

Mum, Nat and Dad - the very best family cheerleaders.

Thank you to my publisher, Jane Morrow, for sending me my favourite email of 2017. For years my community had asked, 'When's a book coming?' I feel so lucky to be able to say, 'It's here!' Thanks to you, Katie Bosher and Madeleine Kane, for making me feel from the get-go that this book was in the very best of hands.

Thanks Nicola Young for being a ninja editor - I felt so lucky to have you as my editor, an accomplished scientist as well as expert maker-of-sense of my at times long-winded sentences!

Thanks to Vanessa Austin, Rob Palmer and Jacqui Porter of Northwood Green for styling, photography and book design respectively, tying everything together into something so gorgeous and approachable - which is exactly how I want these beautiful changes to feel for people!

Thanks to my friends - we place no cages around each other and support each other's actions, ideas and vulnerability in equal measure.

There are so many people whose work I am so thankful for, who inspire me across all the pillars of the Low Tox Life. A few significant ones are Michael Pollan, Joel Salatin, Annie Leonard, Alice Waters, Stephen Sinatra, Ron Ehrlich, Jude Blereau, Mark Hyman, Tim Flannery, Michael Antoniou, Nicole Bijlsma, Marc Cohen, Costa Georgiadis, Brené Brown, Clare Press, Brooke McAlary, Bruce Lourie, Rick Smith, Tim Silverwood, Dan Buettner, Sally Fallon, Dave Asprey, Kirsty Wirth, Joost Bakker, Gary Taubes, Nick Ritar and Elisa Song. All of these incredible people are practising examples, in their work and personal lives, of what's good and true, without judgement, and always inviting curiosity and exploration.

Thanks to all of you activists and sustainable-living advocates out there, who are fighting for our planet in the many ways you do. You are brave, you are needed and I have endless respect for your work. I hope we all live to see the day where what is best for our planet is prioritised over self-serving political and big-business interests.

Finally, thanks to the Low Tox Life community. We are a happy throng of many thousands of conscious, caring, judgement-free people who value that different strokes work for different folks but that real food, simpler personal care and home options, and a low tox mind work for us all. There's absolutely no way this book would have existed without you. Thank you for being here.

I can feel the music coming up and the curtains starting to close (I always wanted to give a Grammy Awards speech!), so I shall leave it there.

INDEX

Published in 2018 by Murdoch Books, an imprint of Allen & Unwin

Murdoch Books Australia
83 Alexander Street
Crows Nest NSW 2065
Phone: +61 (0)2 8425 0100
Fax: +61 (0)2 9906 2218
murdochbooks.com.au
info@murdochbooks.com.au

Murdoch Books UK
Ormond House
26–27 Boswell Street
London WC1N 3JZ
Phone: +44 (0) 20 8785 5995
murdochbooks.co.uk
info@murdochbooks.co.uk

For Corporate Orders & Custom Publishing, contact our Business Development Team at
salesenquiries@murdochbooks.com.au.

Publisher: Jane Morrow
Editorial Manager: Katie Bosher
Design Manager: Madeleine Kane
Designer: northwoodgreen.com
Project Editor: Nicola Young
Photographer: Rob Palmer
Stylist: Vanessa Austin
Production Director: Lou Playfair

Text © Alexx Stuart 2018
The moral right of the author has
been asserted.
Design © Murdoch Books 2018
Photography © Rob Palmer 2018

Extract on page 242 reprinted from *A Pebble for Your Pocket* (2001, 2010) by Thich Nhat Hanh with permission of Parallax Press, Berkeley, California. www.parallax.org
Every reasonable effort has been made to trace the owners of copyright materials in this book, but in some instances this has proven impossible. The author(s) and publisher will be glad to receive information leading to more complete acknowledgements in subsequent printings of the book and in the meantime extend their apologies for any omissions.

Disclaimer: The content presented in this book is meant for inspiration and informational purposes only. The purchaser of this book understands that the author is not a medical professional, and the information contained within this book is not intended to replace medical advice or meant to be relied upon to treat, cure, or prevent any disease, illness, or medical condition. It is understood that you will seek full medical clearance by a licensed physician before making any changes mentioned in this book. The author and publisher claim no responsibility to any person or entity for any liability, loss, or damage caused or alleged to be caused directly or indirectly as a result of the use, application, or interpretation of the material in this book.

A cataloguing-in-publication entry is available from the catalogue of the National Library of Australia at nla.gov.au.

ISBN 978 1 76063 192 5 Australia
ISBN 978 1 76063 439 1 UK

A catalogue record for this book is available from the British Library.

Colour reproduction by Splitting Image Colour Studio Pty Ltd, Clayton, Victoria
Printed by Leo Paper Group, China

Important: Those who might be at risk from the effects of salmonella poisoning (the elderly, pregnant women, young children and those suffering from immune deficiency diseases) should consult their doctor with any concerns about eating raw eggs.
Oven guide: You may find cooking times vary depending on the oven you are using. For fan-forced ovens, as a general rule, set the oven temperature to 20°C (70°F) lower than indicated in the recipe.
Measures guide: We have used 20 ml (4 teaspoon) tablespoon measures. If you are using a 15 ml (3 teaspoon) tablespoon add an extra teaspoon of the ingredient for each tablespoon specified.

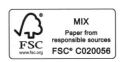

The paper in this book is FSC® certified. FSC® promotes environmentally responsible, socially beneficial and economically viable management of the world's forests.